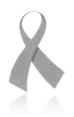

This book is dedicated to the resiliency of the human spirit and to the power of inspirational words.

Y0-AGR-624

PUBLISHER: *Thrivers Publishing LLC*
              P.O. Box 2040
              Lebanon, MO 65536

FIRST EDITION

Cover book design by American Breast Care, LP

Printed in the United States of America

ISBN 978-0-9768995-1-8

Faces *of* Inspirati n

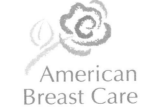

American
Breast Care

www.americanbreastcare.com

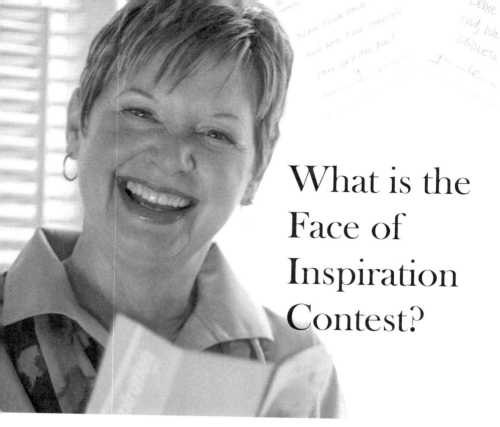

What is the Face of Inspiration Contest?

What is the Face of Inspiration contest?

The Face of Inspiration contest was created by American Breast Care to inspire, uplift and honor breast cancer survivors across the U.S. Since 2011, ABC has selected a breast cancer survivor each year to be the Face of Inspiration. This contest gives one woman the special opportunity to share her inspirational quote and journey with thousands of survivors.

How can I enter?

Breast cancer survivors are encouraged to visit their local mastectomy store to submit an inspirational quote and post it on the *Inspiration Wall* poster. The *Inspiration Wall* poster can be found at any participating mastectomy retailer. At the end of the calendar year, one survivor's inspirational quote will be chosen from the retailer's *Inspiration Wall* and submitted to American Breast Care for consideration. Once all of the entries are received, ABC will choose the top three submissions to be voted on by the

ABC®

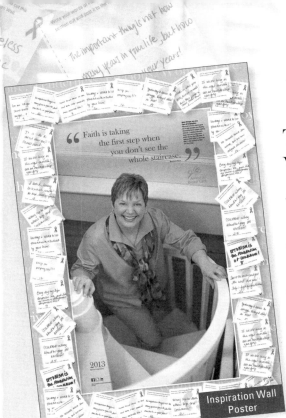

Inspiration Wall Poster

The Inspiration Wall can:

- Provide a spiritual place for survivors to share their inspirational words
- Be a gathering place for survivors, each with a breast cancer story to tell
- Inspire hope in the newly diagnosed
- Allow women to tell their story and feel empowered

public via an online poll at www.americanbreastcare.com. The winner of the contest receives an all expenses paid trip to Atlanta, Georgia for her and a guest, a spa visit, makeovers, glamour photoshoot and so much more!

What is the Inspiration Wall poster?

The *Inspiration Wall* poster serves as a place where survivors can gather to post words of inspiration, hope, love and encouragement.

Why should I enter?

Being the Face of Inspiration gives you the incredible opportunity to share your breast cancer journey, connect with other survivors and inspire women all over the U.S. You never know how sharing your words of inspiration and hope can encourage the newly diagnosed.

Faces *of* Inspirati🎗n

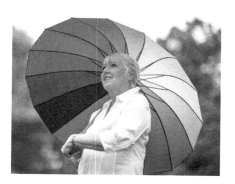

2014 Face of Inspiration
Marge Barnhart
Living for Today..........Page 16

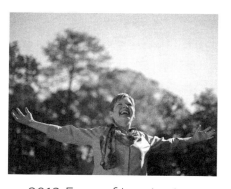

2013 Face of Inspiration
Margo Johnson
Steps of Faith..........Page 76

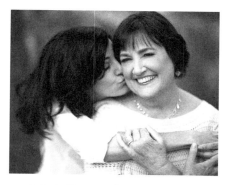

2012 Face of Inspiration
Trudy Smith
Be Brave..........Page 116

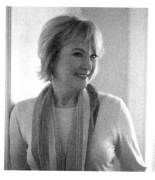

2011 Face of Inspiration
Elizabeth Wagner
The Gifts of Life..........Page 130

Contents

Chapter 3 ~ Faces *of* SUPPORT **47**

Chapter 4 ~ Faces *of* COURAGE **63**

Chapter 7 ~ Faces *of* JOY **109**

Chapter 8 ~ Faces *of* LOVE **119**

Dear Friends,

When someone touches our life, they are not forgotten. These touchstones can make the difference in having the fortitude to move forward on what may seem like the most daunting time of our life. Nothing replaces compassion and the loving touch from someone who cares, or from someone who has been in our shoes.

It is because of three perfect strangers who had been in my shoes and who reached out to me in my time of darkness that changed my life forever. These women had all survived breast cancer decades beyond expectations. Their words lifted me and redirected my journey. I was able to face my life with new found strength and vision. To this day, I feel gratefulness beyond words how they each in their own way lifted my spirit from that dark place.

It would be a decade before Breast Cancer Wellness Magazine would come to be, but I always knew I wanted to give back to others the way *Kay Troutman, Mary Johnson* and *Evelyn Renner* helped me. The journey of publishing has been an extraordinary personal experience because I continue to witness the magnificence of the human spirit, and specifically about the power of coming together to change and uplift the world, one woman and one family at a time. I love bringing together the inspiring messengers of hope and survival to others through the magazine.

Those with the most impact and who have touched my life are my family and friends, breast cancer survivors and mastectomy fitters. When my fitter, Sybil, turned me around to see my new silhouette in the mirror, I was renewed, I felt restored. I left the shop a different woman than when I walked in! The special touch that fitters give to breast cancer survivors are why they are my heroes.

Behind the scenes, American Breast Care works to bring value, beauty and excellence to the products that touch a breast cancer survivor's life. It is also their desire to make a different type of difference with their *Inspiration Program* and that desire is what brought this book to life. It has been a pleasure working with ABC and each of the amazing individuals in this powerful book who shared their messages with us.

I hope these stories will touch your heart and fill you with renewed inspiration, hope, and love. We invite you to share this book with others. We never know when it will be the touchstone someone else may need that day.

Kindest regards,

Beverly Vote
Publisher, Breast Cancer Wellness Magazine

Dear Reader,

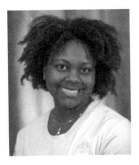

When ABC decided to launch the *Face of Inspiration Contest* and the *Inspiration Program*, we did not know what the initial response would be. We did know that we wanted to create a movement within the breast care community that would ultimately ignite a spirit of inspiration from one breast cancer survivor to another. The *Inspiration Program* was designed to position the local lingerie boutiques, pharmacies and hospital waiting rooms as a gathering place known as the *Inspiration Wall*. The *Inspiration Wall* is where words of inspiration, hope and encouragement can be posted and exchanged among breast cancer survivors.

Being the conduit for this exchange has unveiled this lingering need for a dialogue between survivors in non-traditional places. We tend to think that this type of conversation only exists in the circle of support groups or behind closed doors, but we can see that is changing. It is becoming more common for women to "disrobe" their worries, concerns and anxieties in the fitting room. And even more so, patients are looking to other survivors to find commonalities among each other. The *Inspiration Wall* acts as the hotspot, gathering place or starting point where conversations can begin. Our goal is to start the conversations that happen after; after the initial diagnosis, after chemotherapy, after radiation and even after breast surgery.

At the start of every Inspiration Season, I am reminded of the power of words. Words have the ability to create, change and shape the microcosm we live in. For me, it is simply amazing how a single word of inspiration can influence the present, alter the future and erase past disappointments. After reading the submissions that poured in from women and men from all walks of life, ages and stages, I was truly touched by the many different stories and journeys that stemmed from one common thread — HOPE. It amazes me how resilient the human spirit can be. In times of darkness and loneliness, one word, one touch, one gesture can be the small light that leads to the end of a dark, and yet for many, a bittersweet journey.

I am not a breast cancer survivor, but I have been embraced by this book. What makes this project so special for me is that the words were brought to life by the photograph of each contributor.

After reading this book, I realized that gratefulness is not always a natural response in times of trials and difficulty, but when faced with what looks like an insurmountable situation, you become mindful of those pieces in your life that you once overlooked. The journey of life can be a difficult one, but it is the repeated act of resilience which separates humans from all other forms of life. As you read this book, I trust that you will continue to cherish life and all the beauty that comes with it.

Erika Anderson
Marketing Manager, American Breast Care

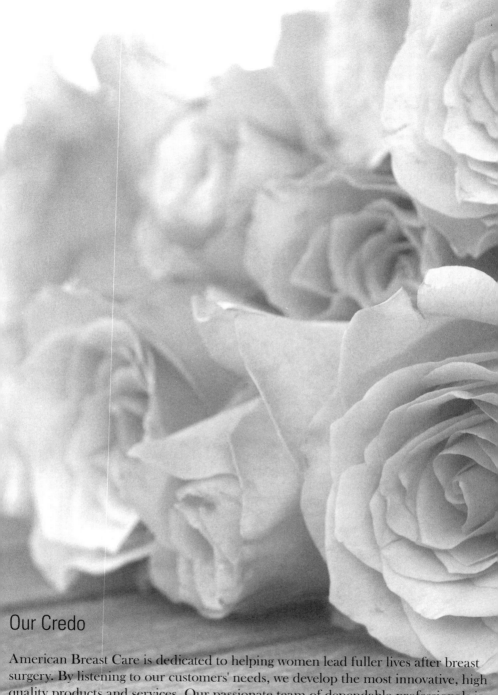

Our Credo

American Breast Care is dedicated to helping women lead fuller lives after breast surgery. By listening to our customers' needs, we develop the most innovative, high quality products and services. Our passionate team of dependable professionals is committed to earning the trust of our customers and the confidence of the women we serve.

Dear Friends,

Many survivors still know very little about the people behind American Breast Care, a leading supplier of after breast surgery products. When we opened for business in 2003, we set out to create a company that listens. By listening to the women we serve, we remain true to the company's core value. Our main goal is to create a collection of products and services that help women lead fuller lives after breast surgery. And over the years, we continue to keep that mission as the basis for all of our decisions.

We are a dedicated team of men and women continually motivated by the common goal of helping women lead fuller lives after breast surgery. That's important. At the beginning of her journey there is a wealth of support to carry her all the way through, but what about life after surgery, when the body she used to know has changed. ABC wants to help when she finds herself in that moment.

When asked to publish *Faces of Inspiration*, we thought that it would be a natural progression for the company. For the past three years, ABC has sponsored the *Face of Inspiration Contest* and *Inspiration Program* within the breast care community. This new endeavor has given us the opportunity to see the power of inspirational words.

We hope that this book will serve as a tangible tool that will enhance the bonds between breast cancer survivors. Think of this book as your personal *Inspiration Wall* — overflowing with hope, faith, love and beauty. May this book anchor the hope of the newly diagnosed and reaffirm the joys treasured by a longtime survivor.

If this is your first experience with American Breast Care, "Hello, it is truly a pleasure to meet you."

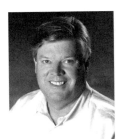

Jolly Rechenberg
Chairman and Co-CEO,
American Breast Care

Jay Markowitz
Co-CEO,
American Breast Care

2014

Face *of* Inspiration: *Marge Barnhart*

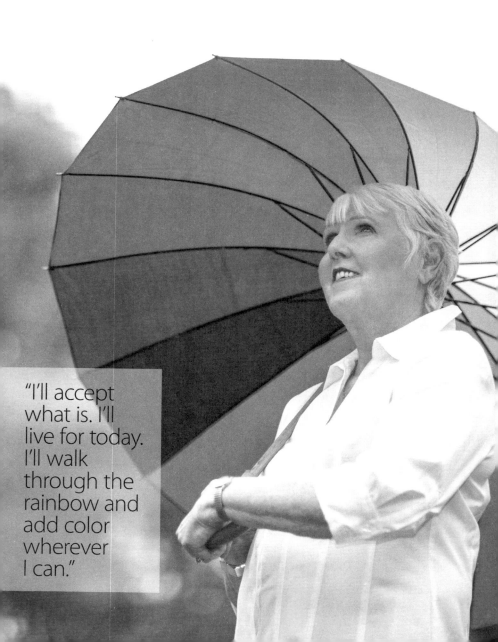

"I'll accept what is. I'll live for today. I'll walk through the rainbow and add color wherever I can."

Living for Today

The following accounts of Marge's breast cancer journey were excerpted from her book, Journey Unknown: Focusing on the Emotional Aspects of Cancer, Mastectomy and Chemotherapy.

In 1987, at the age of 46, I was diagnosed with breast cancer. I underwent a modified radical mastectomy, followed by six months of chemotherapy. To help ease the emotional and psychological burden of the disease and its treatment, I penned poems and sketched artwork. My book, Journey Unknown, is a chronological compilation of these inspirational pieces.

For 46 years I was healthy and energetic, never able to appreciate the struggle of many who endure constant pain and illness. For almost two years, I was a patient in physical discomfort and emotional turmoil. I was dependent on the medical community. I was scared. My emotional state was in turmoil, with many lows and few, if any, highs. My doctor suggested I view chemotherapy as a preventive measure, like the insect spray used in a bed of flowers. That imagery helped me. The loving support of many people carried me through this period.

In a counseling session, I was reminded that I don't need to understand life. I simply choose how to live it. Obviously, I did not choose cancer. Many of the days when I was under the influence of chemotherapy drugs, I questioned if I was capable of controlling my thoughts and emotions. However, I was able to make many decisions along the way. I gradually became aware that as time passed and I "moved on," the focus on cancer diminished and new aspects of my life unfolded.

I've quit fighting. Because I've given up? Given in? No. It's more like giving over, giving way. Too much is outside my control. I'll accept what is. I'll live for today. I cannot add one day to my life. I'll do what I can for the moment. I'll walk through the rainbow and add color wherever I can.

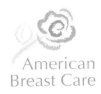

American
Breast Care

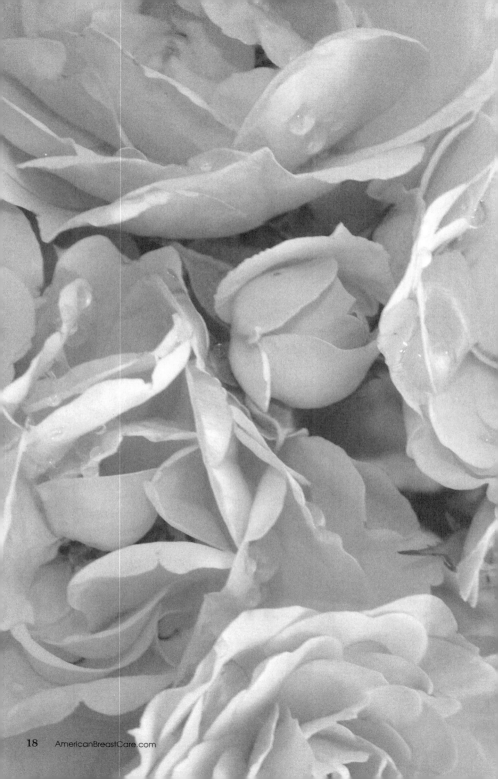

Chapter 1

Faces *of* Hope

"Hope is sweet-minded and sweet-eyed. It draws pictures;
it weaves fancies; it fills the future with delight."
– Henry Ward Beecher

American
Breast Care

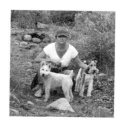

Now I See Blessings

BY CAREY BANNISTER

"Change is for the good."

Eight years ago, I was diagnosed with breast cancer, got a divorce and my dad died. It was a hard struggle, managing the medical schedules, treatments and side effects. My heart hurt that my husband had become vacant to help me, always busy when it was time for my treatments. My dad died suddenly three weeks after I told him that Jay and I were getting a divorce, but I knew Dad approved of the divorce.

I am not a personality to have pity parties, but I certainly didn't understand the harshness and unjustness of my life. But my searching for answers ended when my deceased mother came to me in a dream and whispered the words, "change is for the good" How could divorce be for the good when I was lonely? How could losing my breasts, hair and almost my life be for the good? How could losing the one person who loved me most be for the good? From that dream, I challenged myself to find and to accept the blessing of each day and this transformation of thought changed my life for the better. Now I see blessings, they are everywhere.

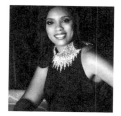

What Can Be Done Today

BY CRYSTAL BROWN-TATUM

"Never feel guilty for taking care of YOU first. You don't want to regret it later."

In 2007 at the age of 35 I was diagnosed with stage IIIa triple-negative breast cancer. Based on charts and outcomes I was given three to five years to live. Although I never accepted or embraced this news, I realized that my mortality was imminent.

As I approach my seventh year without incident of recurrence, I reflect on so many things. First and foremost, I always think of the beautiful women who have lost their fight against breast cancer. As one light is dimmed, I choose to carry the torch higher. My spotlight is powered by their legacies.

I took full accountability for a late stage diagnosis. I waited eight months to see a doctor about the lump in my armpit region. Since I simply did not know better, I made it a purpose and mission to educate women about early detection. Women tend to put aside their own personal needs to care for others but in the end, if we aren't in our right state of mind or health, we are not giving our loved ones our best.

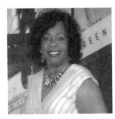

What Matters Most

BY CHERRIE BRICE

"I survived the story by keeping the faith and hope of survival."

It is important to know there is life after breast cancer and that it is important to surround yourself with positive people. If you are a religious person, pray for yourself and ask others to pray with you and for you. Know that you are not alone. Ask your oncologist if there are support groups in your area. Be active in the groups when you find one. Talking about what you are going through helps you to understand that you are not alone.

By establishing in my heart what my top priorities are, and knowing how important each of these priorities are, my decision making becomes easier every day and keeps me from being distracted and interrupted from things that are not best for my well being. I survive the storms of life by keeping the faith and hope of survival.

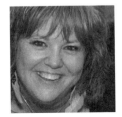

Got Some Living to Do!

BY SANDY CALLIN

"Worry is like a rocking chair. It gives you something to do but gets you nowhere." – Chinese Fortune Cookie

When I was going through my cancer battle (I never capitalize the word cancer) I started a blog. Most of my family is in Canada and I'm in Florida and when I chat with them on the phone, I didn't want it to be cancer talk. I just wanted to find out how everyone's doing, what's the latest funny thing Abby said or sport Cameron was playing... that kind of thing. One day I posted that I was worried all the time that "I have cancer-itis" I said. Later that day I opened my Chinese fortune cookie and it said "Worry is like a rocking chair. It gives you something to do but gets you nowhere." When I got onto the computer later that day, my oldest son had posted the exact same words from the Chinese fortune cookie in response to my post!

So, that has been my motto ever since. Set a timer for 10 minutes and then give your "worry" 10 minutes. Concentrate on it; go to those horrible places that your mind takes you, but when that timer goes off, STOP. No more worrying; after all, you've got some living to do!

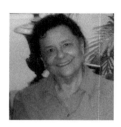

Live, Laugh n' Love

BY CHERI CARRUTH

"Live well, laugh often, and love much!"

Breast cancer forced me to see a more candid view of my present life. I quickly realized I was not alone; many have shared this heartwarming journey with me.

After retiring as a physical education teacher, I owe much of my recovery to the reenacting of a game where the underdog wins. I finally gave myself permission to "suit up, play the game and win" when the odds were not in my favor. I am continuing to play, but have altered my goal to include the game of life.

I am now at a new place within that life since my April 2005 diagnosis. I am still healing, still adjusting, and still living. I still believe in hope, however, I have added some life-changing words to my everyday vocabulary: LIVE well, LAUGH often, and LOVE much!

I always remind myself there is more than one recipe for happiness. But the one I have resolved to count on: LIVING, LAUGHING and LOVING are the main ingredients for living an inspired long, purposeful life!

Stir them well, mix them often, and enjoy them much more.

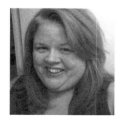

My Stage IV Journey

BY KIMBERLY DAFFORN

"Hope is important."

Being diagnosed with stage IV breast cancer turned my world upside down on December 30, 2006. At that time, most of us weren't sure I would pull through. As my usual stubbornness took over, I went from being wheelchair bound due to the extreme pain to walking on my own and back to work in five months.

This ongoing journey has taught me so much:

I have learned to look for and dwell on the positive. Friends are very important. It's easier being the patient than being the caretaker. Clinical trials are very important for those living with any disease and those that may develop a disease in the future. In a clinical trial, you will ALWAYS get the best of care. Chocolate is good. I might have known that before I got sick, but it's still important. It's okay to ask for help. Most people want to help, but don't know what you need. You cannot fight this disease alone. HOPE is important. Without it we have nothing to live for.

As I continue to live my new normal life with cancer, I reflect on how much hope is out there for those living with advanced breast cancer.

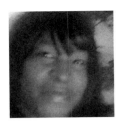

What Kept Me Going

BY PAMELA DUBOSE

"Always look forward."

Hello Fellow Sister and Brother Survivors. My name is Pamela DuBose. I was diagnosed in April 2006 and it has been eight years and counting. I believe in living life to its fullness.

I try not to let anything or anyone one get me down. To be truthful the only ones who really know what we go through are ourselves and God.

Listen to your body, it tells you what you need and how much you can endure. Do not be afraid to ask for help from family and friends; they want to be there for you in anyway they can because they love you.

I had two lumpectomies and seven weeks of radiation. My last day I danced on top of the treatment table and left there with a smile on my face ready to face the world head on. My words of encouragement for those of you who are at the beginning stages of your treatments are that your days will get better and always look forward and never back, keep a positive outlook and make plans for your future. That is what keeps me going.

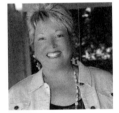

Faith, Hope and Love

BY KIMMIE DURHAM

"Hope anchors the soul." — Hebrews 6:19

As a third-generation survivor, I "grew up" with breast cancer. My journey began in uteri in June of 1958. At age 67, my maternal grandmother was diagnosed with metastatic breast cancer of the left breast. She had a radical mastectomy; which in 1958 was radical! She was cut from her left wrist up her arm across her left chest and another incision stopping at her collar bone. Granny used Kleenex inside her bra... no prosthesis for her! She lived 16 years and remained cancer free when she died at 83.

My Mom received her cancer diagnosis in 1978 at age 52. She celebrated her 35th year of survivorship on December 15, 2013!

On a beautiful Georgia spring day in April 1997, I felt a lump in my right breast while showering. I was only 38. I am now a 17 year survivor and am grateful for each day.

As a third-generation survivor, I am strengthened as my grandmother and mother were with faith, hope and love.

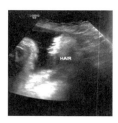

I'm 34 Weeks Pregnant

BY SARA ERZEN

"Life itself is the miracle of miracles." — *George Bernard Shaw*

I'm 34 weeks pregnant with my third daughter. At 21 weeks, I was diagnosed with stage IIb invasive ductal carcinoma that had metastasized to my lymph nodes.

Next week will be my last treatment before I deliver my daughter. She's thriving.

I have done amazing through the chemotherapy treatments. This cancer diagnosis has been a strange blessing in many ways. I credit my unborn daughter with my life because I would not have insisted on further examination if it were not for her.

We had our bi-weekly growth ultrasound today, and my baby looks perfect. She has a full head of hair. My doctor said it's about an inch long which is longer than mine! She is my miracle.

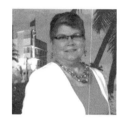

Paying Hope Forward

BY JANET FREDRICK

"There is no wrong way to perform an act of kindness."
— *Catherine Ryan Hyde*

I was given the book called *"The Dash."* It's about a look at our life from the time we are born until our dying day. After finishing the book, a friend of a friend was diagnosed with stage IV cancer. I gave the book *"The Dash"* to this individual to give him and his wife some hope and good thoughts as he goes through the journey of cancer treatments.

While he was receiving his treatments, his wife was in the waiting area reading the book but she was called to the treatment area to be with her husband.

She accidently left the book on the table. When the wife returned to the waiting area to find the book, someone else was reading it. After a while, she went back again to retrieve the book but this time it was in the hands of another reader.

I believe this book was at the right place, and who knows how many it gave hope to.

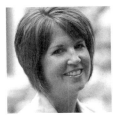

Go Beyond Treatment

BY HEATHER JOSE

"Once we accept our limits, we go beyond them." — *Albert Einstein*

I was 26 when the doctor told me to get my affairs in order. That was 16 amazing years ago.

Initially I wanted nothing more than to survive and I put my entire focus on doing just that. I was all in. *Every Day We are Killing Cancer* became my mantra. Building a strong body and destroying cancer cells one decision at a time, I moved from Survivor to Thriver, acutely aware of the fact that I was made for more, relishing life and the ability to fully live it.

I found that survival was merely a starting point and that cancer was the catalyst to pursuing the life intended for me to help others heal. This has led me to my purpose and passion of empowering women of any age, stage, or phase to Go Beyond Treatment. You can do it, we can help.

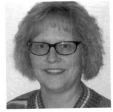

Best Friends

BY KAREN KMETZ

"We cannot change the cards we are dealt, just how we play the hand." — *Randy Pausch*

My sister and I had drifted apart, as siblings sometimes do, even though we live in the same city. Maybe it was the seven year age difference, or our busy lives, but we talked occasionally and saw each other at family gatherings. But when I was diagnosed with stage IV breast cancer, we bridged the gap between us. She came to every doctor's appointment, chemo treatment and all of my scans.

When I craved a particular meal during chemo (which wasn't often), she would make it — especially our mother's lentil soup. Two years later, she helped me through my mastectomy, even staying overnight in the hospital with me. My sister has been there every step of my six year journey through the land of metastatic breast cancer. She calls me every day and has taken me to several conferences to learn about new treatments.

I can never thank her enough for being there when I needed her the most — and for being my best friend!

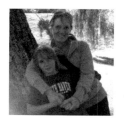

A Spark that Whispers Softly

BY SARAH LEARMONTH

"Sometimes the strength within you is not a big fiery flame for all to see; it is just a tiny spark that whispers ever so softly 'You got this, keep going.'"

I'm 33 and I was diagnosed with metastatic breast cancer to my lungs and bones in June 2013. I was first diagnosed with breast cancer when I was 24 in 2004.

Anytime I faced a hardship, had stress about an upcoming medical test, anxiety over my treatments, or the moments I just felt defeated, I would repeat: *You got this, keep going.*

On the days that it felt it would take a miracle to face the day, I would remind myself to get up, dress up and to fight for my dreams. It was simple but it helped. I felt better by putting on some mascara and lipstick and it helped me to have a reason to be up. Just doing something nice for myself first thing in the day helped me focus on what I wanted to accomplish, which some days, what I wanted to accomplish was to simply get through the day without thinking about my illness.

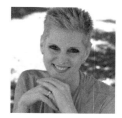

From This Moment On

BY TAMBRE LEIGHN, MA, CPC, ELI-MP

"As our days proceed into our ever-growing destiny, I believe we can truly create something from nothing at every moment of our existence." — Gary Charles Wissner, Hodgkins, 1964~2001

After my late husband's diagnosis, even through the darkest times, Gary insisted we find a way to experience as many extraordinary moments as possible.

Gary wrote this quote in the last birthday card he gave me before cancer took him. He believed, with all his heart, it is in our power to create the moments that make up our lives even when we're facing circumstances we didn't necessarily choose. He didn't see destiny as something written in stone long ago but as a living legacy created in the moment out of the thoughts and actions we choose to take.

As our days unfold before us, our legacy takes shape and is filled with moments in which we can either create nothing lasting or the most meaningful, impactful actions that make the greatest difference for both ourselves and for others. From this moment onward, what will you choose to create, no matter what the challenges you are facing? It is... always... a choice.

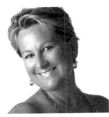

Living Well Fills My Heart

BY LORI C LOBER

"God can inject hope into a absolutely hopeless situation."
— *Mark Evans*

In April 2000 I was diagnosed with stage IV breast cancer. I went through a period of shock that produced many mixed thoughts and emotions. Cancer can certainly be life-threatening but it does not necessarily have to be life-ending, even at stage IV.

Positive thinking will provide the foundation for inspiration and guidance, to always stay the course and to never give up. Understand that negative and even heart-breaking news can fuel you throughout your struggle to beat cancer. I realized that even the most helpless situation can be reversed and transformed into power.

Hopelessness can be countered by conviction, control and the realizations that the mind is extremely powerful and sometimes it is possible to achieve the seemingly unimaginable. "Cancer wants to kill me" — I had to put this thought out of my mind.

Hopelessness does not exist in the mind of a positive thinker, so I got rid of it. Instead, I came to realize how much in control of my life I could be, regardless of the presence of cancer in my body. The daily reality of living with and fighting cancer offered little hope, but taking control and becoming determined to live and live well, filled my heart with hope.

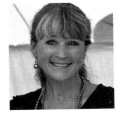

Stay Positive with Laughter

BY WENDY MCCOOLE

"Laughter is an instant vacation." — *Milton Berle*

I learned a lot from my mother who battled breast cancer four times. She was an amazing woman. She definitely had her glass EMPTY moments and knowing how that felt on the receiving end I made the choice early on to stay as positive as I could. When I went through breast cancer I did everything in my power to keep a sense of humor, but what my mother did was remarkable! A few years after she had a mastectomy she did a short stand-up comedy bit at a charity event and it was hysterical! She talked about how she was now a "pididle" and asked the audience what the singular of cleavage was. She talked about her first prosthetic and how it kept crawling up her neck like an alien creature. She shared how she would walk up to a wall to make sure both her "boobs" touched at the same time and how her new(er) prosthetic was "as perky as ever" while her other breast sagged to the floor. The audience adored her as did we. The message here is that it's relieving (and necessary) to feel sad sometimes, but laughter truly is the best medicine!

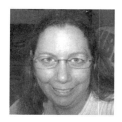

Laughter Is Healing

BY PAULA MCCOY WILLIAMS

"Laughter brings strength"

I was diagnosed on June 5, 2006 with stage II breast cancer at the age of 37. I was shocked and devastated by the diagnosis as breast cancer did not run in the family and I never expected to have cancer.

I was mad at God for the longest time for having me go through this. After awhile, I realized that if I had to forgive God and rely on him as he was the only one that would see me through. One thing that helped me through my journey was maintaining a sense of humor. I realized that if I took everything too seriously all the time, I wouldn't be able to make it through. I had to laugh at the toughest things, such as losing my hair. I couldn't bring myself to shave it before I started chemo so I lost it all less than a week after my first chemo treatment. At first I had a good cry about it and then I told my mom that I wouldn't need a costume for Halloween, I could go as Baby New Year. As hard as it was to laugh about it, I found that laughter was healing and it gave me the strength I needed.

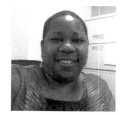

Celebrate Anew

BY MARA PARRISH

"Kicking cancer by God's grace, love and mercy."

My annual physical in October 2012 included a breast exam which didn't reveal any concerns in my breasts. However two weeks later I felt a lump in my left breast that I assumed was related to premenstrual changes. The lump didn't go away and within two weeks, it actually got larger. I went back to my primary care physician who was shocked that it appeared out of nowhere. I had a mammogram, ultrasound and biopsies on both breasts. I received my results on January 4, 2013; my left had invasive breast cancer and my right breast was pre-cancerous.

The following week was full of tests, an ECG followed by port installation and a plan of action to treat breast cancer. I had chemotherapy for two months, bilateral mastectomy without reconstruction and radiation.

I kept smiling that I only had to deal with a few minor hiccups during treatment.

I went back to work with a new normal to celebrate and am now loving life to the fullest!

Her Legacy Lives On

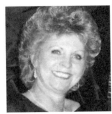

BY BONNIE PHELPS

"Each one of us can make a difference. Together we can make change."
— Barbara Mikulski

My beautiful sister Barbara died four decades ago at the age of 29 with breast cancer. She was eight years older than me. She was diagnosed at the age of 27 one year after her fourth child was born. By the time she was correctly diagnosed, the cancer had significantly advanced. I think back how different it was then; you didn't talk about cancer, you didn't discuss feelings, there were no support groups or Pink Sisterhood. She was so young. Today I still wonder how did she feel, what did she think, was she scared? I wish we had talked about it.

She had a wonderful personality and was very talented. She played the piano and had a beautiful singing voice. She played the piano at my wedding.

The changes that have taken place in the years since her death are remarkable. Cancer is talked about and feelings are discussed. There are many wonderful resources that my sister didn't have. Working with the Breast Cancer Wellness Magazine has been a healing experience for me knowing that we are making a difference and bringing comfort to the lives of women with breast cancer, the difference I wish I could have made for my sister.

I Am a 10 Year Survivor

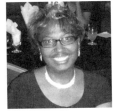

BY LAKENIA ROBINSON

"Cancer is a word, not a sentence." — John Diamond

I'm a 10 year breast cancer survivor. I was a single mom of a 14 year old daughter who was a freshman in high school. I was 39 years old, recently divorced, just purchased my home and on my job for 19 years. On October 14, 2003 while performing my self-breast exam, I felt a lump in my left underarm and testing revealed a lump on my left breast. On November 28, 2003 I was diagnosed with breast cancer. I was devastated and having to tell my daughter was one of the most challenging parts of this experience.

On January 7, 2009, again while performing my monthly breast self-exam, I felt a lump on my right underarm. On January 9, 2009 I was again diagnosed with breast cancer.

My daughter has now graduated with her Bachelors and Masters Degree in social work. Today, I am cancer-free.

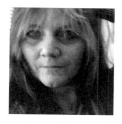

Beginning a New Chapter

BY SHERRIE SARVER

"Where there is no vision, there is no hope."
— George Washington Carver

I was diagnosed October 16, 2013, the middle of breast cancer awareness month. I was laying in my bed at home from work watching a television program on breast cancer when I got the call giving the results of my biopsy. I expected it to come back fine. I was in shock, I could not handle it.

I had a lumpectomy on November 6 which did not provide optimum results. On December 31, I had a bilateral mastectomy. It was a painful experience but I began 2014 cancer free.

I am feeling more like myself and am thankful for the new chapter opening in my life. Thank you God for I know the day will come when my treatments will be completed.

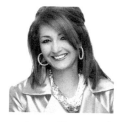

A New Chapter in My Life

BY REGINA SERNA

"Happiness is not something ready made. It comes from your own actions." — Dalai Lama

I was diagnosed with stage II breast cancer in April 2009. After many doctor appointments, two lumpectomies and finally a bilateral mastectomy with reconstructive surgery for a total of five surgeries, I'm cancer free!

My former employer terminated my career in October 2009; their behavior changed once I informed them of my diagnosis during a time I thought they would be most compassionate. Yes I did sue and was successful not only for me but for all who find themselves in similar situations.

I have experienced loss of job, car, savings and finally my home that I loved. It was very devastating and emotionally draining. During this time I gained 45 pounds because I just did not care, I was no longer working out or eating well. The depression was deepening. I applied for a job and much to my surprise I was called a year later for an interview. On December 29, 2013 I moved to Chicago to begin a new chapter in my life and to rebirth the deep happiness that calls my name.

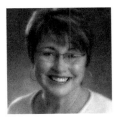

Having the Right Attitude

BY PATRICE SOBCZNSKI

"Whether you think you can or you think you can't, you're right."
— Henry Ford

This is one of my favorite quotes. I truly believe our attitude has so much to do with the outcomes in our lives. I'm certainly not saying that a positive attitude can cure cancer, but I do believe having the right attitude can help you triumph over some of the difficult treatments and side effects.

My mother has always said that "everything happens for a reason." When I was diagnosed with breast cancer at age 37, I wondered if I was meant to be an example that breast cancer can happen at a young age and always hoped that my diagnosis would encourage other women for proper breast screening and self care.

I am a 25 year breast cancer survivor and have worked in the post-breast surgery products industry for 23 years. Cancer is not the worst thing that ever happened to me. Breast cancer brought me to a wonderful career helping other breast cancer survivors. I look at it like I took breast cancer and "turned lemons into lemonade" (another favorite saying).

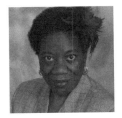

My Faith in God

BY ANNIE RUTH STATEN

"If I can help somone as I pass this way, then my living will not be in vain."

The most important aspect of my 27 year breast cancer journey that I share with other survivors is my faith in God and the blessing of being a Survivor. I encourage you to:

- Wake up every day saying WOW!, I am alive.
- Live life to the fullest regardless of your circumstances.
- Be willing to offer encouragement to other survivors with kind words and a listening ear.
- Share your story from your heart, it may be the spark for another survivor.
- Include a dash of humor and laughter in your daily routine; it is definitely a stress buster.
- If you feel a pity party coming on, have a PRAISE party, sing a song or repeat your favorite scriptures.
- Surround yourself with positive people.
- Always know that you are God's miracle and He has left you here for a reason.

To God be the glory.

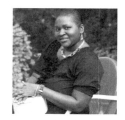

Light at the End of the Tunnel

BY TANYECIA STEVENS

"Don't watch the clock. Do what it does: keep going." — S. Levenson

On February 2012 I found a lump in my left breast. I thought to myself maybe it's nothing but a pulled muscle. I ignored it and went on with my life until July when I felt two rigid masses under my arm. They felt like golf balls. I didn't have insurance at the time. I waited until open enrollment to be on my husband's insurance. I went in for an ultrasound and then a biopsy. November 20, 2012, I was diagnosed with stage III breast cancer at age 33. I also found out I was six weeks pregnant and had to make the choice of keeping my unborn or terminating my pregnancy and starting treatment right away. I underwent six months of chemotherapy, bilateral mastectomy and seven weeks of radiation. I don't know where I found the strength to pull through and today I am NED (no evidence of disease). I just want women to know there is light at the end of the tunnel. Never give up, not matter what life throws your way.

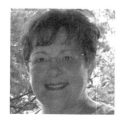

Don't Waste the Miracle

BY PAT NEELY STEWART

"Keep busy building memories with family and friends."

I was diagnosed with breast cancer in 1999. I celebrate the joys that I have been blessed to live since my diagnosis, two mastectomies, and chemotherapy. Today, I am an advocate for breast self exams as well as regular professional mammography. Knowing our bodies is important for survival.

Along the journey, I gained so much both in awareness and perspective while in the midst of extreme sickness, unreal fatigue, losing my hair and realizing I had a 70% chance of surviving five years. Life is good and full of gifts that we sometimes don't see except in the darker days. One of my greatest blessings in life has been my deepened relationship with Jesus Christ who is my constant companion for life.

My journey has taught me so much and at the top of the list is that in our every day lives, the people we encounter all have needs and we have the resources to help meet those needs. Encourage is to inspire with courage, spirit, and hope. Every thing we need to encourage others lies within our own hearts.

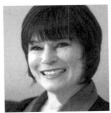

Strength in Humor

BY LOUCINDA SULLIVAN

"But I've bought a big bat. I'm all ready you see. Now my troubles are going to have troubles with me!" — Dr. Seuss

An evening on Google compelled me to rush to my doctor clutching pages of evidence. I knew at my core the innocent-looking spot on my breast was about to hijack my life.

Not now! Please cancer, let me get organized first.

Nope.

I dug deep for strength, leaned on my husband, and together we pulled out humor. Laughter would help my body, and my loved ones, heal.

Remember the song Hot Blooded by Foreigner? Here's my version:

Well I'm PET scanin', check it and see. Injected isotopes inside of me. Come on baby don't make me glow green like that. I'm PET scanin' PET scanin.'

My husband threated to write on my bald head with permanent markers. A Tic, Tac, Toe board. "This End Up." A poem, written in a spiral so he could spin me in a chair to read it.

Humor got me through months of treatment. You can do this, too. Smile, and make cancer wonder what you're up to.

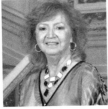

My New Mantra

BY EUNICE WALKER

"With God, all things are possible!"

Diagnosed with breast cancer in 1987, I chose to have a mastectomy. After losing a sister to breast cancer plus two brothers and my 18 year old son to traffic accidents, I realized my breast was the least of the losses I had suffered!

In 1988 I had my other breast removed and had reconstruction. There were complications. In 1990 it was removed and my right arm was paralyzed. I was given little chance for recovery of my arm. I refused to accept that! One month later I left the hospital with a huge apparatus on my arm and hand.

After months of therapy, help from friends, my mother and so many people praying for and encouraging me, I was playing tennis again!

Early on I realized that I was granted the privilege of survival. My personal inspirational quote "Survival is a privilege; recovery is a choice" became my mantra. With a positive attitude and faith, I believe we can recover from most things. "We are in charge of our attitude."

I don't have natural breasts, but if I felt any more like a woman, you probably wouldn't like me at all!

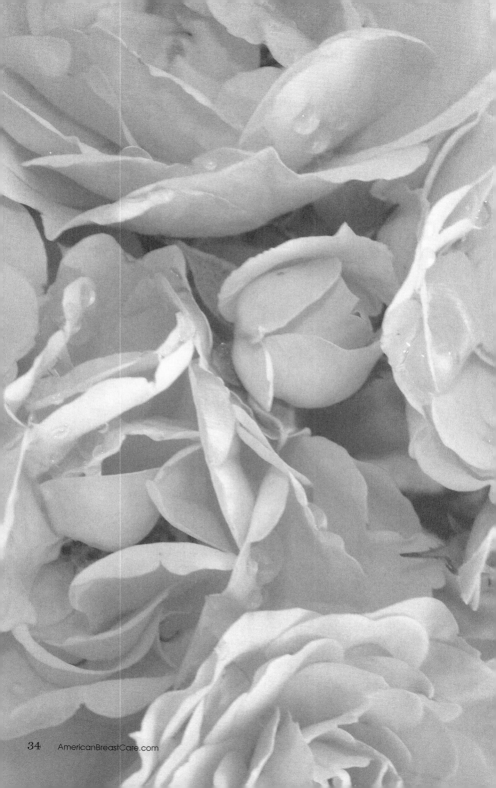

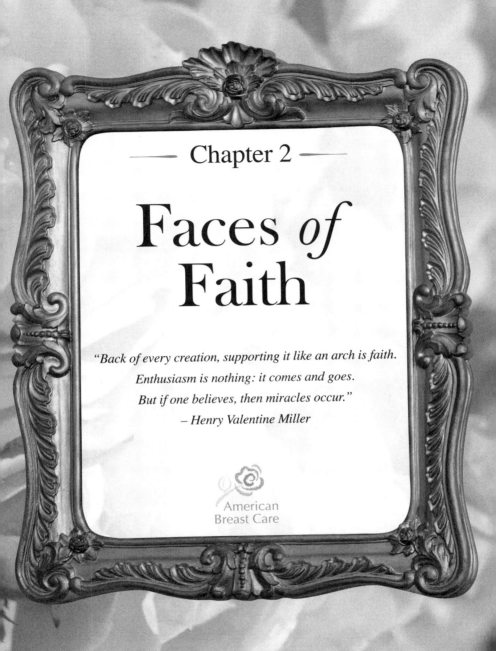

Chapter 2

Faces *of* Faith

"Back of every creation, supporting it like an arch is faith.
Enthusiasm is nothing: it comes and goes.
But if one believes, then miracles occur."
– Henry Valentine Miller

American
Breast Care

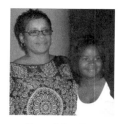

Starting Anew

BY LEATTA ASBERRY

"Never let go of faith, the battle is won."

Dear Mr. Cancer,

No one deserves to live like this; you have forced your way into my life! I want you to know that you will not control me or my life because I refuse to let that happen!

I don't love you and never will.

None of my friends or family like you either so I am divorcing you. You can have the house, the cars, and all the money, just let me go! No form of love for you has ever lived here and never will!

It's time for us to go our separate ways, I need to start anew, I command of you!

It is time for you to bow out gracefully because this is one fight you will not win! Jesus is representing my case.

Sincerely, Ms. Asberry

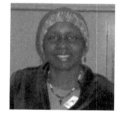

I Changed My Style

BY VANESSA AUSTIN

"God will not leave you or forsake you." — *Deuteronomy 31:8.*

God will not leave you or forsake you. How do I know? Well, I am a two time cancer survivor — breast and ovarian. Without God in my life, I would not have any hope. God is my comforter, my healer, and my deliverer. And "God is our refuge and strength, a helper who is always found in times of trouble," Psalm 46:1.

Since being diagnosed, I have changed my style of life which includes eating healthy foods, staying positive, enjoying the goodness of life, and pursing my passions of reading biblical material, writing books and poems, handcrafting jewelry and greeting cards, and embroidering handkerchiefs.

Being an artist and a writer helps me relax my mind and my body. In addition, my talents and gifts help me stay sane and stay focused on God. Plus I read, pray, and meditate on God's Holy Word, knowing that God's Word heals and God's Word is true.

Lastly, I have come to realize that God operates in His timing, *not* ours, so you *must* keep on praying and *never* give up, because "God is mighty in battle. Let Him fight your cancer!"

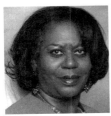

How Did I Do It?

BY VANESSA BARRIENTZ

"Every great movement of God can be traced to a kneeling figure."
– D. L. Moody

I am a two-time breast cancer survivor. The first time was in 1999. The treatment I had was lumpectomy, chemotherapy, and radiation.

I prayed and asked God to give me strength, because I did not feel as if I could take the last chemotherapy treatment. Every treatment made me sicker and sicker. God answered my prayer and I did take the last treatment.

Everything was fine until 2013. I was again diagnosed with breast cancer. I had a mastectomy. Thank God no other treatment was recommended.

My faith in my Lord and Savior, Jesus Christ, and the support of my husband, family, and close friends is the only way I got through breast cancer twice.

I know God has something more for me to do. My work on earth is not finished. I thank God for my husband, family, and friends who helped me get through so much. My sister calls me her Super Hero. In spite of everything I have gone through, cancer is only one thing, God keeps giving me the strength to do what He has for me to do.

Put your trust and hope in Jesus! He will give you the strength you need also.

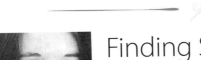

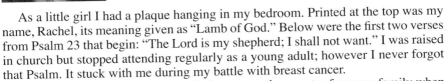

Finding Solace

BY RACHEL BROOKS POSADAS

"The LORD is my shepherd; I shall not want. He maketh me to lie down in green pastures: He leadeth me beside the still waters." – Psalm 23:1-2

As a little girl I had a plaque hanging in my bedroom. Printed at the top was my name, Rachel, its meaning given as "Lamb of God." Below were the first two verses from Psalm 23 that begin: "The Lord is my shepherd; I shall not want." I was raised in church but stopped attending regularly as a young adult; however I never forgot that Psalm. It stuck with me during my battle with breast cancer.

I was in my twenties, single, and living across the country from my family when I was diagnosed. Going to daily radiation sessions and follow-up oncology appointments left me feeling alone and I wished there was someone to hold my hand through it all.

Just when the sense of loneliness got overwhelming, I'd think of Psalm 23 and remember that I was never really alone as God was always there with me.

These verses gave me comfort and helped me through one of the most difficult times of my life. I still find solace in them even now as a survivor for over 10 years.

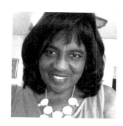

Not Once, But Four Times

BY YVONNE CISCO

"Now faith is the assurance of things hoped for, the conviction of things not seen." — Hebrews 11:1

In 1987 I was diagnosed with terminal breast cancer. I was told to get my affairs in order for my remaining three months. I believe my miraculous recovery was because of the power of prayer. There were family, friends and even strangers from across the United States to Jerusalem who began to pray with me and for me. I had always believed in prayer but this was an up close and personal experience. I am a living testimony to the real power of prayer. When hope was gone, prayer stepped in, not once, but four times. My prayers and the prayers from others have empowered my actions and stopped me from letting fear over take my life. I had surgery and a year of chemo and 36 rounds of radiation. I continue to have medical examinations every four months. After my recovery, I established a goal to teach others to give back to those in need by providing a helping hand of love, charity and compassion through volunteering. I'm still here because God hears and answers prayers. How awesome!

My SHERO

BY ANDREW KEITH COLLINS

"We are the hero of our own story." — Mary McCarthy

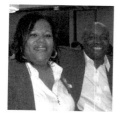

Seven years ago my wife was diagnosed with breast cancer. When she decided to pray and give her body to Christ, she woke up the next morning and it was like she didn't have anything. From that point, she never cried, never worried, never complained and never thought of giving up. She made up her mind that she was going to fight this thing and I joined the fight with her. I went to every chemo and radiation appointment with her.

When she lost her hair, I decided until it grew back, and because I was already bald-headed, that I would shave off my mustache. As long as you put God first in your life and lean on Him, there is absolutely nothing you can't accomplish.

Since retiring from the military after 30 years, I have never served with a trooper with more heart than my wife. Hope, Faith and God are what we had to get us through.

Make Your Heart Happy

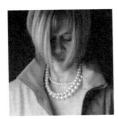

BY HEIDI FLOYD

"Do everything in love." — *1 Corinthians 16:14*

I am not a 'survivor' of breast cancer. I am a patient and will always be a patient. While I live with, rail against and push away from this disease every day, it does not mean it rules my life.

I was diagnosed while pregnant. My cancer journey was difficult and terrifying every single day. I had three beautiful little daughters, a husband getting his masters degree and absolutely no time whatsoever for cancer. Friday chemo was followed by Monday ultrasounds to make sure the baby was doing okay, to make sure his little heart hadn't stopped beating, and that he was still growing. There was not one moment that didn't involve me constantly praying that he would somehow survive this ordeal.

My oncologist told me that my life has been abbreviated; what I choose to do with my fragile time line should reflect things that only *truly* matter. The stress caused by irrelevant minutia remains a huge factor in my treatment. How does one, I asked my beloved doctor, do things that only truly matter?

His reply changed my life: "Do what makes your heart happy? I don't mean to avoid the mundane or monotonous. We all have to do things that aren't fun all the time. As a matter of fact I am fairly certain that what you find rewarding would reduce many people to tears. You need to lend comfort to those in need, those who are going through cancer. Find people who need you, and embrace them. It will hurt you, your heart will break when they simply can't get better. When they can't be healed and need to talk to someone about their pain at 2 a.m, you should be on the other end of the phone. It will be such a hard thing, this life, but you need to do this."

So I did. I sought and found people in need. I've prayed with them and for them, screamed with joy at great test results via text in England and wept with a young widower in Australia as he said goodbye to his wife. I've been to more funerals than I can count, but ache with regret at the ones I simply couldn't attend. These people have changed me, and I've been honored to know them.

I found a new tumor in 2011, which resulted in a complete mastectomy among other surgeries. I've found incredible, amazing joy as well. My family gives me endless reasons to be thankful. My son, healthy and strong, walks with me and his sweet sisters to school every day — a feat I never dreamed I'd accomplish.

So no, I am not a survivor. I'm not angry at the word, not upset about my diagnosis or bitter about my constant companion named cancer. I prefer to see it as a tag along on my life journey, and I'm bound and determined to help as many people as I can for as long as I'm allowed. Faith and hope, that's all I've got.

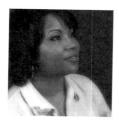

Living a Life of Purpose

BY ADRIENNE GORDON

"I will lift up mine eyes unto the hills, from whence cometh my help. My help cometh from the LORD, which made heaven and earth."
— Psalms 121:1,2

God truly is amazing! In 2004 I experienced hearing the words, "You have breast cancer." The diagnosis of ductal carcinoma in situ (DCIS), an early-stage of breast cancer, was my kind of initiation to a new life of service to God. I write with you in mind as I reflect on how I felt when I was first diagnosed and had to undergo a mastectomy. My advice to you is develop your faith in God and find a way to serve Him instead of worrying about the "what wills" and the "what ifs." Focus on living a life of purpose from this day forward.

I remember hearing messages like "It's only a test" and "God wants to show you something." Ten years later, I am still here to say that those messages came straight from God through the people He had placed in my life to talk me through the darkness. God is real and He is a Healer! Embrace this opportunity to get to know Him for yourself and always look up!

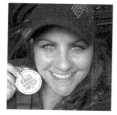

Making Every Moment Count

BY KIRSTEN GREENFIELD

"The Lord has not only restored my health but everything in my life. I stand on His promise of healing and a plan for my future."
— Jeremiah 29:11

In 2007, I was a mother of three boys and a wife of 14 years. I was diagnosed with stage IV breast cancer and life as I knew it changed instantly. Why was it not caught earlier?

I had symptoms for three years but was told repeatedly that I was too young for breast cancer and they were explained away as something else. It has been a very long and difficult journey. I chose to have a bilateral mastectomy and endured almost three years of chemotherapy, radiation and more surgeries.

In 2009 during my treatments, my husband unexpectedly passed away from a heart defect that had gone undetected. Shortly after his death my best friend passed away from her five year battle with breast cancer.

Only by my faith in Jesus did I make it through such difficult times. I have been in remission for close to five years now. I have remarried a wonderful man with three beautiful girls.

I live every day as if it were my last, making every moment count.

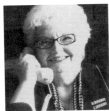

35 Years Later

BY JEAN HOLLINGSWORTH

"For I know the plans I have for you." — *Jeremiah 29:11*

One morning back in the 70's, I caught a graphic television segment about self-breast exams. Instinctively I followed the directions — raising my right arm and placing my hand on my breast. There, my fingers felt a small lump.

In those days, the surgeon would put you to sleep and you would either wake up with a small incision or a radical mastectomy. I woke up to hear the "c" word. The recovery was slow and painful but our friends and family showered me with love.

Looking back, I remember asking if God really had plans for me.

But then, the world became so beautiful, the colors so vivid, and my faith grew stronger as God revealed "His plans for my life." I didn't just "happen" to see the TV show and discover the lump. Early detection saved my life!

Today, 35 years later, I am cancer free! I lived to enjoy our four children, seven grandchildren, and 10 great grandchildren who make every day like Christmas. I am blessed to have the sweetest husband for more than 60 years.

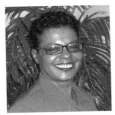

One Goal in Mind

BY MONTEZ (TEZ) Y. HOLLINS

"When you treat a disease, first treat the mind." — *Chen Jen*

In November 2010, three months after a normal yearly mammogram, I felt a large ball under my arm while showering. On January 14, 2011 the diagnosis was triple negative breast cancer that had spread to my lymph nodes. After the initial shock, tears shed together with my husband and alone — in that order — it was hard to grasp the fact that I had breast cancer. The fear I felt is indescribable. All I could do was pray for strength, courage and a positive attitude to do what I had to do to become well. With my faith and mind right, I learned everything about this cancer to prepare myself for the journey ahead.

I leaned on all my sources of inspiration — my faith in God, the love and support of my husband, family and friends (near and far) who rallied around to raise me up in my time of need. In addition, all the women I met at my doctors' offices inspired me immeasurably because collectively the goal was to beat breast cancer!

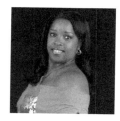

A New Voice

BY LASHUNA JACKSON

"My Faith gave me the strength I needed to defeat the breast thief."

I had just become a newlywed when I was diagnosed with breast cancer. Just hearing those words was shocking. All I could do was pray! I recall looking up to the sky and saying "Okay God, you helped me find this lump, I'm trusting you to heal me." My husband and daughter walked this journey with me every step of the way; we even participated in a breast cancer walk together. I realized this journey was chosen for me; I was not going to let cancer make me a victim, but help me to inspire others to fight. God gave me strength, courage, new friends and a VOICE, a voice that will help others in my situation know they're not alone and can win! I have chosen to live my live my life like a camera, take the negative and turn it into something positive. Turn your journey into inspiration for others.

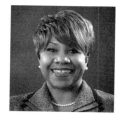

My Faith Sustains Me

BY VALERIE D JACKSON

I can do all things through Christ which strengthens me.

I was shocked at the news that I had breast cancer. I was in pain from the lump I complained about for two months. I was alone. I called a coworker and asked her to cancel a seminar I was hosting because I was scheduled for surgery the next day. She told me to focus on my health and not the job. She picked me up, cooked me dinner, and then took me dancing to keep my mind off of my medical circumstance. She said she didn't want me to be sad or alone after hearing my diagnosis. Now that's a noble friend.

I have faced many challenges with cancer. I was literally cut by having 14 cancer related surgeries, experienced eight aggressively harsh chemo treatments and 70 radiation treatments. Through it all, it's been my faith in God that sustained me. It was also the steadfast love and support from family and friends who encouraged and motivated me to endure my cancer journey not once, but three times.

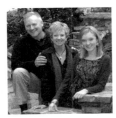

Unfailing Strength

BY JULIE KAYS

"God will either shield you from suffering or give you unfailing strength to bear it."

Where do you find the strength to carry on? I am asked that question quite often. When I was 13 my mother died of breast cancer, the next year I lost my grandmother to cancer. At 16, I was diagnosed with ovarian cancer, and at the age of 32 I was diagnosed with breast cancer. I had both breasts removed before my husband and I celebrated our first anniversary.

My daughter, our only child, was diagnosed with brain and spinal cancer two years ago. At the age of 15 she underwent brain surgery followed by over a year of chemotherapy. She continues to struggle with the effects of this terrible disease.

All I know for sure is that without faith, my family and I would be stumbling in the dark. One of my favorite quotes that gives me comfort and peace in times of fear and uncertainty is "Have no fear for what tomorrow may bring, the same loving God who cares for you today will take care of you tomorrow and every day. He will either shield you from suffering or give you unfailing strength to bear it. Be at peace, then, and put aside all anxious thoughts and imaginations." — St. Francis de Sales.

I find my peace in faith.

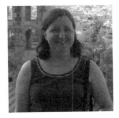

Seven Years Cancer Free

BY MARCIA MEHRTENS

"Choosing an attitude of faith will release peace out of your spirit and into your soul." — Joyce Meyer

The nurses at my oncologist's office said they wished they could have made me the poster child for chemo, as I always had a smile on my face and faced it with such determination. My belief in God is strong and with the power of prayer and my amazing family and friends by my side, I knew that I could beat cancer and I did. I am happy to say that I am seven years cancer free and living every day to the fullest.

Some people may think of cancer as a curse, but for me it was a blessing in disguise. I took a leave of absence from work while I was going through treatments which gave me time to spend with my aging parents that I otherwise would not have taken.

For anyone facing this diagnosis, I say smile and never lose faith.

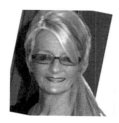

That Day On

BY MARLYS OISTAD

"Never look back."

I received the first breast cancer diagnosis in 2000. I was 56. I had one breast removed; I wanted the other removed, but they would not do it for me.

I received my second diagnosis of breast cancer five years later. I had the other breast removed. I went thru 18 months of chemo and six weeks of radiation.

I was devastated the second time and really just wanted to go to bed and stay there. However, when I shared that with my daughter, she cried and said she hated God. That was an awakening for me. I told her to go home and get her walking shoes on and that I would be there to join her. From that day on, I never looked back and just praised God for all the blessings I had received from Him. He is my strength and my hope. I knew that I had to forge on for my family. He gave me everything I needed to do it.

I am still here. I am 69 and doing great! Praise the Lord.

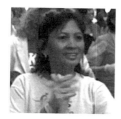

Humility and Faith

BY LEAH SALMORIN

"There is always light."

Humility and faith in God are two lessons I learned from cancer.

Through some government workers, I learned to be humble, diplomatic and forgiving of their insensitivity. I also forgave my then-landlady who practically kicked me out for fear of being responsible for me because my family didn't live close.

My faith in God comforted me; with him beside me, nothing is impossible. I kept a positive attitude despite all adversity because God held me close to his side. I am blessed because I was well taken care of. My doctor, nurses and staff were very accommodating and courteous.

Through my journey I was able to give back too. I worked as a hotline volunteer and patient navigator and made friends with other survivors whose stories inspired me. I learned a lot from my "sisters."

When asked how I beat cancer being alone, all I can say is God fought my battle for me. I believe at the end of the dark tunnel there is always light and I can get through. I am thankful to him for transforming me into a better, stronger person and helping me achieve my highest potential.

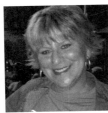

It Will All Be Worth It

BY KERYN SHIPMAN

"I let my faith heal and guide me."

I thought the hardest thing I was going to have to handle in my life was beating breast cancer at 34 and seeing my mom lose her battle from the disease at age 61. I was wrong. The real test came 13 years after my first diagnosis with a new breast cancer battle after just losing my job. I was faced with going through the battle again but this time without either my mom or dad who are both deceased and I had no job. It was the darkest point in my life.

This diagnosis was a real test of my faith. But it is my faith that actually got me through this battle with the beast. You see I had to go through the fear, loneliness and at times feeling of hopelessness to realize that what doesn't kill you does make you stronger if you allow it.

I didn't allow it to break me, I let my faith heal and guide me which it continues to do today. Our hardest times often lead to the greatest moments of our lives. Keep the faith, it will all be worth it in the end.

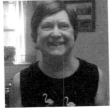

I Didn't Give Up

BY GLORIA WALKER

"I believe that God has a plan and purpose not only for the human race, but for my individual life. — Anne Graham Lotz

At first I was devastated at the diagnosis. My husband had already been through throat cancer. I turned to God and asked why? I realized that I had to let others help me and let go.

It was a difficult treatment journey and many times I wanted to give up and quit. I had many months of being ill and tired.

My husband was a great encouragement to me and my daughter Glorita and grandchildren Emily and Devin always had a smile and hug for me. When my granddaughter Emily went wayward, my family and I prayed daily for her to return to be a part of our lives.

Soon after my diagnosis and prior to my mastectomy my granddaughter Emily came home. My faith in God and the support from my family helped me through each day and on December 12, 2013, I was declared cancer free.

On January 14, 2014, I became a great grandmother to a precious baby girl, Emicree. I know that God had a plan.

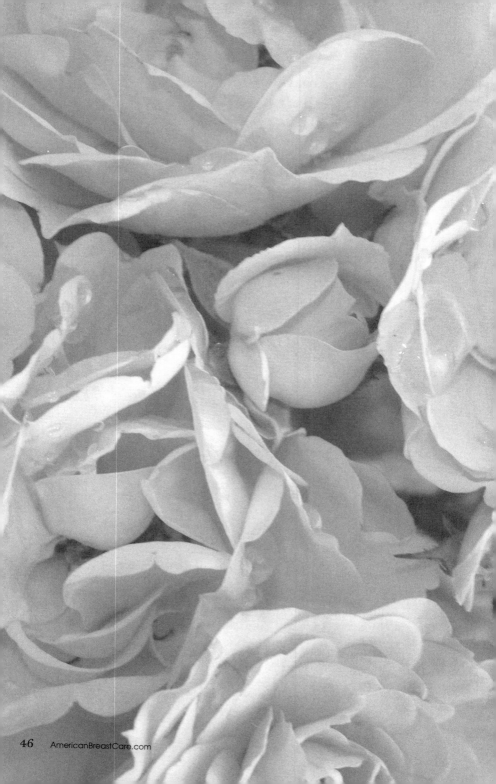

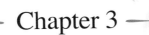

Chapter 3

Faces *of* Support

"Encourage, lift and strengthen one another.
For the positive energy spread to one will be felt by us all.
For we are connected, one and all.
– Deborah Day

American
Breast Care

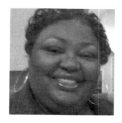

Celebrating 31 Years

BY BEVERLY HUNTER ANDERSON

"To be fully seen by somebody and be loved anyhow — this is a human offering that can border on miraculous." — Elizabeth Gilbert

One morning in April 1983 I was enjoying a long shower with my favorite music echoing through the house. As I soaped my body I remembered this was a great time to do my breast self-exam. I laughed as I thought about the day the health nurse came to my high school when I was 17 to teach us about BSE. My journey back to the past was rudely interrupted as my fingers glided across a small lump in my breast. Rinsing away the soap, I immediately checked for a mosquito bite... no such luck.

After I had a modified radical mastectomy on my right breast and six lymph nodes removed, I begin six months of chemotherapy (no port). I was 26 years old, bald as an eagle, one breast, sores in my mouth, bruised arms from blown veins, and dark nails. I was a hot mess! Nevertheless, I have never felt more loved. Family, friends, coworkers, and church family surrounded me with love and prayed me through the storm. Thirty-one years later I am a Survivor!

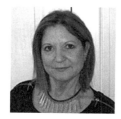

Life is Rich with Purpose

BY LORI BARAN

"One person can make a difference, and everyone should try." — John F. Kennedy

I am a stage IV metastatic breast cancer crusader. I have approached the fight against breast cancer with zeal and enthusiasm. One thing I know for sure, is that we cannot survive without the people who have already traveled the road that we are on and who know the journey. Part of the healing process is giving back, and thus my life as an advocate has evolved over the past few years.

You can make a difference by being active for change by taking part in educating others and through breast cancer organizations you believe in. You can share your story in a book, magazine or a blog, and have a voice in the breast cancer research grant review process.

I take an active role in educating newly diagnosed women on integrative ways to get healthy. You must first educate yourself by reading, attending conferences, and joining advocacy groups and advisory committees. You will find that your life is rich with purpose! Don't ever stop trying to make a difference. Let your voice be heard, and I promise that someone will listen and benefit.

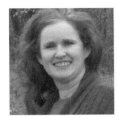

The Golden Rule

BY LAURIE BENNETT

"Do unto others as you would have them do unto you."
— The Golden Rule

My mother's diagnosis of breast cancer brought a new perspective that penetrated the hearts of women in my family and in my community.

I was too young to understand what breast cancer was when my mother was diagnosed but I was at a perfect age to witness the love, support, and heartfelt encouragement that surrounded her.

Because of the level of compassion my mother displays now for generations of breast cancer thrivers, I am inspired to do the same. I have learned to be a better listener and to give both encouragement and a helping hand.

By supporting a woman to arise from a diagnosis of breast cancer and to choose emotions and motions that are full of life bring blessings both for the recipient and the giver. Breast cancer brings the opportunity to improve on the blessings we already have by being a better person, a more caring family, and generously giving more to others.

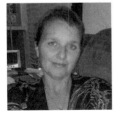

Celebrating Cancer Free

BY SARAH BULLER

"The more you praise and celebrate your life, the more there is in life to celebrate." — Oprah Winfrey

My story started in January of 2013. My youngest child was about to have her first birthday. I found a lump in the left side of my breast one day. I finally got up the courage to ask my mom to check and see if she also could feel it. She has been a nurse for over 30 years and I knew she would be honest.

When she felt it and told me I needed to get it checked, I started worrying. I am a single mom of three beautiful kids and had no insurance! I didn't know where to start. Luckily there was an organization locally that funded my care, and got me insurance to pay my medical bills. I have completed my medical treatments including getting my implants on March 11, 2014. What a way to celebrate one year cancer free!

Stronger

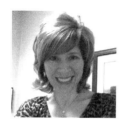

BY KRISTINA COHN

"Some of your greatest pains become your greatest strengths."
— Drew Barrymore

I was diagnosed with DCIS at 41 years old. I didn't have any symptoms or family history, but simply because my doctor suggested I go for my first mammogram during my yearly physical. I was nervous, and not knowing what to expect, I pondered whether or not to keep the appointment. Little did I know that this would begin a roller coaster ride of emotions that I never would have suspected.

After a few mammograms, an ultrasound and a biopsy, I will never forget the call or the words "the biopsy tested positive for cancer." Why me? I don't smoke, I eat healthy and I exercise three to four times a week.

Exactly three weeks after my news, both my Mom and our cousin were diagnosed with breast cancer also.

After multiple surgeries between us, as well as our individual treatment plans, we are extremely grateful and proud to say that we are SURVIVORS three years later!

Our faith and family helped us to persevere and get through the bad days to finally realize that breast cancer did not define us, but rather, it only made us stronger!

Comfort and Support

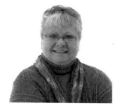

BY DIANE DAVIES

"Reaching out to help others on their journey has ultimately provided me with comfort and support as well."

My six-year-old granddaughter asked me if I knew the "S" word. The "S" word I thought? At least I had dodged the "F" word bullet.

The terrifying "c" word, however, could not be avoided in 2004 when I was diagnosed with breast cancer. Hearing the word cancer connected to my body was shattering to say the least. Suddenly there was no place to go to dodge what I took to be a death sentence. No longer listening to what was being said, I began to plan my funeral.

That was when a number of "F" words came into play to see me through the journey and carry me across to the other side stronger, wiser and grateful for having made the trip — faith, family and friends.

Of all the lessons I learned from my cancer, these are the most meaningful: Love comes in many different ways and forms. Life is good. Life is precious. An attitude of gratitude is important. A gracious receiver is just as important as a generous giver. By reaching out to help others, you ultimately help yourself.

By the way, the "S" word in question was "stupid." Not what I had in mind at all.

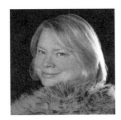

Prepare to Move On

BY GAIL DUSCHA

"Grief is in two parts. The first is loss. The second is the remaking of life."
— Anne Roiphe

Since my diagnosis, I assist the newly diagnosed in any way possible. Many just need to see a survivor to affirm to themselves that they too can survive, others need advice, direction or a shoulder to cry on.

I encourage women to acknowledge their sadness, grief, fear, etc. give "it" its due course but do not live there. Limit your time when you indulge in it and be strict with yourself to end it and then move on.

I put my diagnosis and all of its baggage in a box, and put it on a shelf. Sometimes that box falls off the shelf and the contents spill out. I give "it" its time then gather it up and put it back in the box and onto the shelf. In the beginning it falls off that darn shelf quite a bit, but as time goes on it falls off less and less.

If you allow cancer to beat you in your head or destroy your spirit, then no medical treatments will be able to help you.

Now who is bringing the wrapping paper to this pity party?

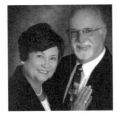

Look for the Rainbows

BY ANNE ERICSON

"When life's storms pass you by, go look for God's rainbow."
— Mary Alice Morrow

Mary Alice was my grandmother, simply Ma to me. My cousin and I spent our summers with Ma. Whenever we had a thunder storm, we would hide behind the bed. Later, when the storm had passed, Ma would say "The storm has passed, now go look for God's rainbow."

In 1974, days after my 31st birthday, I had a radical mastectomy. My surgeon reported that "everything looks clear, no sign of cancer." In other words... "the storm has passed, now go look for God's rainbow." That was 40 years ago.

After my surgery, I had a strong desire to help women look and feel better about themselves after breast surgery. Since 1985, I have worked as a breast care specialist with a wonderful company that manufactures breast prosthesis and surgical bras.

My husband Eric and I have five sons, and three grandchildren. Eric has always supported me and my work. He's treated me like I am the Love of his life, regardless of my surgery.

I never see a rainbow that I don't think of my sweet Ma.

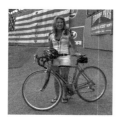

Support Creates a Lasting Memory

BY LIZ FREGEAU

"Never believe that a few caring people can't change the world. For indeed, that's all who ever have." — Margaret Mead

Hi, I am Liz Fregeau. I am from Portsmouth, NH. I am a two time breast cancer survivor. Treatment for my second diagnosis included chemotherapy and a bilateral mastectomy. One month after my treatment ended, I got back on my bicycle for a 163 mile bike-a-thon along with over 5,500 other bikers to help raise awareness and money for an organization that helped save my life.

My favorite and most memorable moment from my 13-year participation in this event occurred in 2010 when my daughters surprised me by meeting me at the finish line when I was bald and worried that I wasn't going to complete the ride. My family's constant support continues to motivate me each and every day to make a difference for myself and current and future cancer patients.

Because I personally know how important support is for survivors, I helped form a support group for breast cancer survivors. It has grown from 10 members to over 700 members strong. The ultimate goal is to help eradicate breast cancer so that others won't suffer.

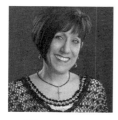

Giving Back

BY ELISA GUIDA

"Life is a gift, and it offers us the privilege, opportunity and responsibility to give something back by becoming more." — Anthony Robbins

Nine months after getting married in 1995, I heard the words "you have breast cancer" that forever changed my life. To cope with the daily medical treatments, I planted plants and flowers in my backyard. That was the beginning of my love for gardening, which I found to be very therapeutic. My backyard became my personal oasis!

In 2008 while attending a Bon Jovi concert with my husband Ed, I thought — why not get famous musicians to donate their used guitar strings so that I could turn them into jewelry or art! With the monies raised, I could help people with breast cancer. That's how the charity that I started was born. Just like the flowers in my garden needed nurturing, breast cancer patients need education, comfort and support.

To date we have provided over 400 gas, grocery and pharmacy gift cards to breast cancer patients. We have also provided medical grants so that women with lymphedema can purchase the garments they need.

Giving back has been my inspiration.

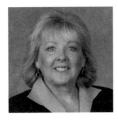

Gentleness Needed

BY CYNTHIA HASKINS

"Nothing is so strong as gentleness, nothing so gentle as real strength."
— St Francis de Sales

I probably know my sister best especially since I read her little pink diary often when we were children. I remember to this day how she bats her eyes when she is nervous and how she holds her fork. It was our memories of our times together that became the medicine that kept this caregiver going. I wasn't the typical day-to-day caregiver. I was a caregiver from afar. We lived more than 1,500 miles apart.

I realized that this was not about me, and nor was it just about her. My sister needed my strength and I needed strength to give to her. Through prayer, it was delivered. This new found strength was greater than ourselves.

On one of my visits to see my sister, she looked deeply into my eyes as she tried on her first wig in preparation of losing her hair from chemotherapy. It was an unspoken moment. The room became quiet. A gentle energy filled the room. Gentle was all that we could handle at the moment. And yet as gentle as the energy was, it brought hope, faith and bravery.

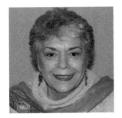

Still Going Strong

BY BOBBI HANKS

"In every community, there is work to be done. In every nation, there are wounds to heal. In every heart, there is the power to do it."
— Marianne Williamson

"It doesn't look good. It's malignant! It's advanced breast cancer with a prognosis of five years!" I remember looking over my shoulder to see who the doctor was talking about. It couldn't be me.

I had a wonderful job at the time of my diagnosis, one that combined my music background and my love of writing. Then one Friday, I went to work and found the doors chained shut. Everyone was so sure I was going to die that they would rather close the business than deal with my impending death. I was left with no health insurance and no income while still in treatment for breast cancer. This inspired me to help create a breast cancer program dedicated to improving the lives of all women. We've served more than 7,000 women.

Twenty-seven years and three different cancers later, I'm still here and going strong.

What was my mantra during the tough times? "I'm too busy to die, it's not in my Daytimer and no other woman will wear my jewelry." Somehow it's worked.

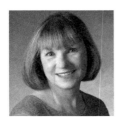

Getting Through

BY ROSEMARY HERRON

"Get through it, then get through to others."

I had long been a nurturer and a caregiver type of person. I volunteered in three hospitals while in high school, then went on to become a nurse. I married, had children and volunteered in schools, church and community. I was used to being the doer, fixer and helper. That changed in 2001 when I was diagnosed with stage II invasive ductal carcinoma and had to endure six months of chemotherapy, a lumpectomy and six weeks of radiation. I experienced complete role reversal and depended on others for help. I just had to find something positive to focus on and adopted "Get Through It, Then Get Through To Others" as my mantra. When treatment was completed, I joined local breast cancer advocacy groups and presented breast cancer awareness education in the community. I wanted women to be aware of their breast health. I also volunteered in the breast clinic of the major cancer center where I was treated, sharing my experiences with newly diagnosed women. Now, one year after a second breast cancer diagnosis, chemotherapy, bilateral mastectomies and recent reconstructive surgery, I am still trying to help others by showing them you can get through it a second time!

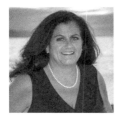

Getting a Second Chance

BY KATHY HOWA

"Get in, detect early, and fight like a giant with the best of attitudes."

Some people don't get a second chance in life after a diagnosis — no matter how hard they fight. When we do, we need to turn lemons into lemonade.

I was diagnosed in 2002 with invasive carcinoma in stage II and went through two studies, surgery, chemotherapy, and radiation.

At the school where I taught, the athletic director and my athletes rallied and helped me start a fundraiser. It began in Utah and has traveled across the United States in softball and is now in all sports, including kids in all grades as well as all levels of college athletes.

Since 2002, the youth have raised over a million dollars for breast cancer research. The foundation is all volunteer based and 100% of the funds go to research.

I have been forever blessed by so many all over the nation and in turn we have taught them about early awareness, giving back to the community through sport, and to be bigger than themselves in life.

I have learned so much about myself, others, and how not to take life for granted.

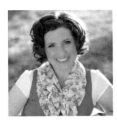

Make All the Difference

BY GINGER JOHNSON

"Oh, my friend, it's not what they take away from you that counts; it's what you do with what you have left." — Hubert Humphrey

I agree with holocaust survivor Viktor Frankl: "When we are no longer able to change a situation, we are challenged to change ourselves."

Breast cancer hit my life when I was 31 years old and five months pregnant. Unable to change the situation, I was determined to change how I would experience it.

In between my treatments I would canvas the community to get prize donations for other cancer patients. Before my infusions began, I would introduce myself to the other patients, sing them a song about how opposition is part of life, then proceed to hand out donated prizes wishing recipients 'Happy Chemo!'

Little did I know that this simple act of service would blossom into what is now a national network connecting tens of thousands of people facing cancer to approved products, services and resources. What started as a way to cope has become an 'oxymoron on a mission' to increase the hope, health and happiness of those facing cancer.

While we can't always control what happens to us, we can choose how we will act in any given situation and that, my friends, can make all the difference. Choose wisely.

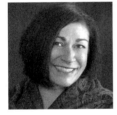

Healing Follows Believing

BY PAM KNOWLES

"Carpe Diem."

I'm Pam Knowles, caregiver to Judy Knowles, 94 who is a two time breast cancer survivor.

What I now have to show for a life excessively touched by cancer is a firm grasp that the present moment IS a Present! I also have a large box of Thank You cards for being there. "Carpe Diem" is inscribed on a silver bracelet gifted from a friend recovering this week. Seize the Day. You must!

Ovarian cancer haunted my gene pool three times, so sitting with my Mom-in-Law for her first diagnosis of breast cancer, I was the epitome of ignorance but nonetheless was present to provide wonderful loving support. Six years later at her second diagnosis, I had been around the block. Now with three close friends/thrivers, I told Mom's doctor to STOP talking and let Mom catch her thoughts. Then asked the question everyone should carry on a note: "What do we need to know that we have not asked?" Doctors become amazing resources from that point. Healing follows Believing — in your doctor, your treatment plan, your family, and your higher power.

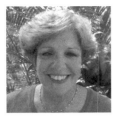

A Blessing to Help Others

BY CONNIE LARKIN

"The joy that you give to others is the joy that comes back to you."
— John G Whittier

My name is Constance Larkin and I am a licensed massage therapist.

Early in 2013, I got a call from my younger sister Janice. She had been diagnosed with breast cancer and she needed my help. Part of her treatment included removing 28 lymph nodes from her underarm. Janice also went through chemotherapy and radiation.

Janice asked me to go back to school to learn more of what could be done for lymphatic care after breast surgery. I found the best school for this specialized field. This training provided me opportunities to help other women facing the same situation my sister faced and to educate women on the benefits of proper lymphatic drainage modalities after breast surgery.

It has been a blessing to be able to help others.

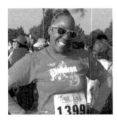

Pink Advocacy

BY SARITA JOY LITTLEJOHN

"In helping others, we shall help ourselves, for whatever good we give out completes the circle and comes back to us." — *Flora Edwards*

In 2005 at the age of 36 I was diagnosed with stage I invasive ductal carcinoma breast cancer. After treatment in 2007, I was even blessed to give birth to a healthy baby boy. I retired in 2006 and was able to devote my time to helping other women with a breast cancer diagnosis. I became involved with advocacy and affiliated with several breast cancer agencies. I participated in breast cancer awareness walks to raise money for a cure.

In February 2013, I returned to my dream job as a patient navigator. Helping members of the community navigate their cancer treatment was the ultimate satisfaction. I became active in the gym and altered my diet to incorporate a healthy lifestyle. I even began running and completed my first half marathon.

In July 2013, the cancer was back — stage IV breast cancer. All of the effort I made to help others and arm myself with information was really for my benefit.

Although living with mets is difficult, it doesn't keep me from educating, smiling and thriving!

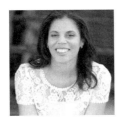

Transform the Suffering

BY SABRINA MAYHEW

"As my sufferings mounted, I soon realized that there were two ways in which I could respond to my situation—either to reach with bitterness or seek to transform the suffering into a creative force. I decided to follow the latter course." — Martin Luther King Jr.

While recovering from my breast cancer surgery, I received a heart shaped pillow to help ease my physical discomfort. It was created by a stranger who wanted to help me on my journey to recovery. I was truly touched by this small gift that gave me emotional and physical comfort in a time of deep hurt and disappointment. Today it reminds me of how a small gift can make a large impact. Reflecting on this, I wanted to share this gift of love and hope with others.

The Angel Pillow Project gathers cancer survivors together who understand the unique needs and challenges women face after a breast cancer diagnosis. Creating the pillows is a way to build community and connect with others. We are nurturing, compassionate, warm, loving and caring. It is empowering to be able to take such a difficult, painful experience and use it to grow a community of survivors committed to helping others through difficult times.

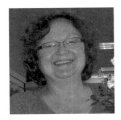

Listening

BY ROBIN MOSHER

"You need to listen to your body because your body is listening to you." — Dr. Phil McGraw

The radiologist's report was that it was probably benign. "Probably" didn't sound very confident to me. My doctor said we'd look again in six months but he wasn't worried. I was. My aunt was dying of breast cancer. Another aunt was a two-time survivor.

When I asked for a biopsy he said there was probably no need but he knew I needed the reassurance. The surgeon reminded me that 80% of biopsies are benign and that there would be a scar. A scar didn't bother me, cancer did.

I think it was harder for my surgeon to give me the cancer diagnosis than it was for me to hear it. When we listen to our bodies we unconsciously prepare ourselves. From the moment my surgeon said "I'm so sorry," I knew that listening to my body had saved my life.

The most rewarding thing for me is when I give one of my patients a hug and she tells me that she feels reassured after meeting with me. You see, God put me in this place at this time for this reason. As a mastectomy fitter for over 25 years I've met thousands of breast cancer thrivers, listening to their stories is as important to me as it is to them.

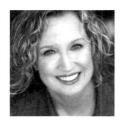

The Beauty of Each Day

BY JAN PING

"To me being beautiful is how I share my gifts in my life and how I honor what each day brings me."

Imagine working in Hollywood with some of the most acclaimed beautiful people in the world. Hello, I am Jan Ping, an Emmy winning professional make up artist to the stars. You would recognize the long list of celebrities who are my clients. But an additional avenue was added to my life when I was diagnosed with breast cancer in 2004. The diagnosis helped me see my life's calling in a new way. It was then that I realized on a deep level that I wanted to make a difference for breast cancer survivors and everyday women and help them emphasize their individual beauteous best.

There were times after breast cancer that I was filled with self doubt and I somehow believed I wasn't enough. The changes that came along with breast cancer made me realize these are unhealthy beliefs and they hinder us from seeing the best in ourselves and in others.

When I help women see their beauty, it is such a powerful healing moment for them and for me.

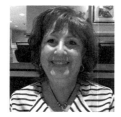

Still Surviving, 32 Years Later

BY ODELL SAULS

"A woman's attitude is important."

When I was first diagnosed, I cried. I was only 36 years old at the time and was married with two children. Years have passed and one important lesson I have learned from having breast cancer is this: It is not the worst thing that can happen to a woman.

Through my cancer experience I have been able to help other women who are newly diagnosed. As an R.N., I started a support group for breast cancer patients. It was a wonderful time of sharing and learning.

Breasts seem to be the ultimate physical quality in our society but a woman's attitude is just as important. A woman can wear a prosthesis, get reconstructive surgery, and wear sexy clothes. And most men can deal with the "new" you fairly well.

After reconstructive surgery, I shared the "new" breast appearance with other women who were afraid of how their chest might look. They were pleasantly surprised.

Today, I am 68. My breast cancer experience has helped me grow as a woman. I have met some wonderful people and I can face challenges in life and say, "I survived breast cancer, I can survive this too." And so can you!

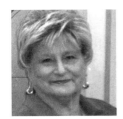

I Live With Gratitude

BY BRENDA POINDEXTER SCROGGINS

"God isn't finished with you yet."

I'll never forget the day! It was November 24, 2008, my husband's birthday—the day I received the call confirming breast cancer. The biopsy doctor had somewhat prepared me by telling me not to be surprised if the report showed cancer. For the first few moments it was TOTAL shock—then tears and suddenly my survivor skills kicked in. I began to think; what should I do first? Which doctor should I use? What treatment should I choose, etc.? Thankfully, I have a loving family who helped support and guide me. I was blessed to have a medical support group that included wonderful female physicians, a breast cancer navigator and caring nurses. I'm happy to say that thanks to my faith in God and the support of great family and friends, I have been able to live most days joyously, with very few sad days! I have met MANY wonderful people along this path; people that I would have probably never encountered if it were not for this diagnosis. Several inspired me by saying, "God isn't finished with you yet," so I try to live each day with gratitude!

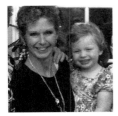

Make It Matter

BY JEAN SOUTHARD

"Hope is the thing with feathers that perches in the soul and sings that tune without the words and never stops at all." — Emily Dickinson

I was diagnosed with breast cancer on February 10, 2009. I have had a series of revelations since then. Some came during that first 24 hours. My family had gathered and it was so quiet... so somber that it felt like a funeral. I reminded them (and myself) that this diagnosis didn't mean I would die today, and that I had life left to live. I had two married daughters, one granddaughter and another due in three weeks. It suddenly became very important to me that my grandchildren remember me. I wanted to make the fear I saw in my husband's eyes disappear. They were my inspiration.

I became very open with people and wanted them to understand it was okay to talk about cancer. I learned to put myself at the top of my list of priorities. I accepted the support of family and friends as they became invaluable in my recovery. Life became something I lived rather than rushed through. I found good in every day, even in bad days. I continue to find that "good" and embrace it. I hope you find the "good" in your day, every day.

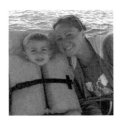

In This Together

BY CHRISTINE TAYLOR

"Compassion is a feeling deep in the heart that you cannot bear someone else's suffering without taking steps to relieve it." — Dalai Lama

At the time of my diagnosis, my idea of what it meant to have breast cancer had one ending. I had watched helplessly as my young aunt succumbed to the disease and I was terrified.

Shortly after my diagnosis a nurse confided that she had breast cancer eight years ago. A friend shared that she was also eight years out of treatment. The woman fitting me for my wig had breast cancer 10 years ago. My yoga teacher was over 20 years out. Everywhere I went I met someone with a wonderful story of survivorship. The care, compassion and words of hope that they gifted me with were exactly what I needed to realize that I could have my own story.

I am now a practitioner who helps women with cancer. I help them improve their quality of life and move their life forward. It is rewarding to now be the face of hope for others. We are in this together. Using your experience to help others is one of the greatest gifts you can give.

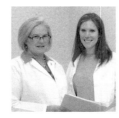

Collaboration

BY IDA TRICE VALAVIK, RN, MS, RNP-BC AND JENNIE MCLAUGHLIN TARICA, MSN, RN, CBPN-IC

"Every woman deserves a caring team."

Every woman deserves a team to help her confront breast cancer. As a Nurse Navigator and a Breast Surgery Nurse Practitioner, we help women begin their healing journeys by assessing each patient's needs and ordering the appropriate diagnostic testing. Taking extra time with every woman to reassure and educate them prepares each for their road ahead. It is our mission that our patients feel embraced and supported as they move forward with their specialists.

We experience the rewards of collaboration between patients and their medical team every day when we witness women having confidence to take control of their disease and no longer be traumatized in fear. Having an accessible, reliable and caring team working tirelessly is how we make a difference every day for the women we serve.

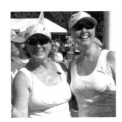

Passionately Pink!

BY VALERIE WRIGHT

"Keep on keeping on!"

I was lucky enough to meet my "soul sista" Teresa Jones at my second chemotherapy treatment. It was her 11th treatment. It was in June 2011. We became the breast of friends and always will be.

Teresa and I have walked together in so many ways, including breast cancer races in Denton, Texas in July 2011 and September 2011 and Plano, Texas in June 2013.

We both embraced our baldness. We know that God brought us together so we could have each other through it all. We are forever grateful. We are proud to be PINK!

Her favorite quote is "Another day, another gift!

My inspirational words are "Keep on keeping on!"

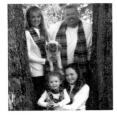

Be the Change

BY BRAD VOTE

"You must be the change you wish to see in the world." — *Gandhi*

Everyone knows the word 'cancer' but not everyone knows how that word will affect you and your family. It all comes down to attitude, positive or negative. It is always your choice to accept it or deny it.

I chose a third option, to ignore it. If I was too busy to be involved, I didn't have to face it. My mother had breast cancer. I am thankful for her willingness to embrace it, fight it, and make a difference in the lives of other women.

As a teenager I didn't know how to help. Twenty-two years later I see and understand the importance of a strong network of caring friends and family. I now understand that my mother did not choose to have cancer, but she did choose to fight it.

I am truly amazed by the thousands of women she has helped with her magazine. She will be the first to tell you that she learned about positive attitude from those who went the journey before her. Her positive choices have changed many lives and more personally, my perspective.

Be positive, be courageous, but most importantly, Be the change!

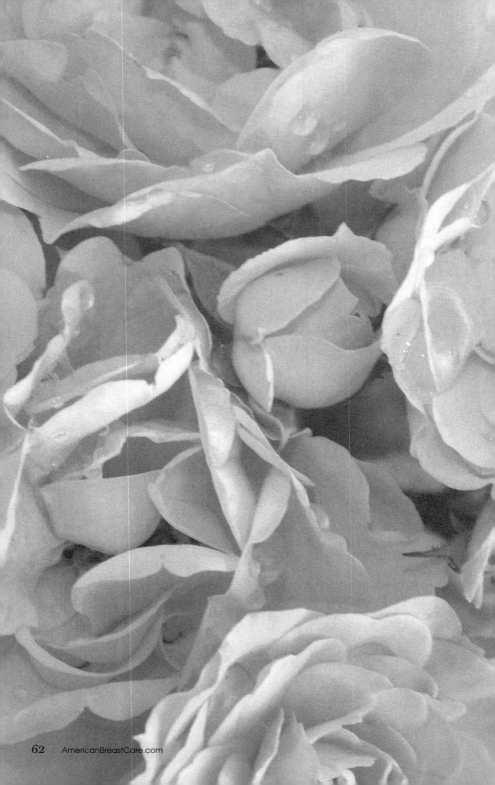

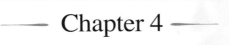

Chapter 4

Faces *of* Courage

"Above all, be the heroine of your life,
not the victim."
– Nora Ephron

American
Breast Care

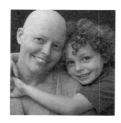

Endure This

BY VICKIE BAST

"With a few great friends and caring doctors, you can get through almost anything."

I was diagnosed with stage III breast cancer in July 2011 which was two years into my unemployment after being laid off in 2009. Needless to say as a single mom with no job and no insurance, this was not the best time to hear the news but then again when is? On August 24 I walked my five year old son to his first day of kindergarten and the next day had a right breast mastectomy to remove a handball size tumor. Surprisingly, I handled the entire process fairly well as I moved from diagnosis to surgery then treatment. I was even able to include my son in the process as I let him use my fresh, bald head as a canvas. Outings to oncologists, chemo, and radiation got me out of the house and fed my mental health with interactions. I also found Facebook very cathartic as I posted the good and bad of what I was going through especially in and out hospitals with double pulmonary embolisms and pneumonia. I discovered with a few great friends and caring doctors you can drag yourself through almost anything.

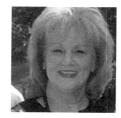

YES, I truly am a SURVIVOR

BY PATRICIA BENTON

"Never give up!"

In 2009 I was diagnosed with stage IIIa breast cancer. This was the hardest thing in my life I have had to face.

Things I learned since having a lumpectomy, chemotherapy and radiation treatments is that ALL things are possible through Christ. NEVER GIVE UP. Faith and grandchildren gave me the will to fight.

As I was ready to participate in my fifth breast cancer fundraising race, my granddaughter Mallory and I were standing in front of the grandstand. I stepped out to walk towards my husband and my tennis shoe caught on the barricade and I fell. As the paramedics worked on me, I thought "this cannot be happening to me." As I got up, I looked into Mallory's eyes. I had to show her that I was a survivor. After the bleeding stopped, I asked my husband if he would go buy me a clean shirt. I was going to walk for all the women who are going through what I had to endure! I NEEDED to make this walk. I did it with two black eyes, a nasal fracture, and a fracture in my right arm.

Don't Let Fear Stop You

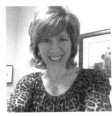

BY COREY CALLIGANO

"You gain strength, courage and confidence by every experience in which you really stop to look fear in the face." — Eleanor Roosevelt

I looked fear straight in the face in September of 2012 when I was told I had breast cancer. I went through five months of chemotherapy, had a lumpectomy with 18 lymph nodes removed under my left arm, six and half weeks of radiation, one year of herceptin and now I will be on tamoxifen for the next five years.

At 30 years old, with three small children, I was scared of the outcome. There were so many days I just wanted to give up. The treatments didn't save my life, my children did. Without them, I probably would have never got out of bed. I survived this horrible experience, and now I'm thriving from it!

Everyday should be taken as a gift, learn something new, enjoy a beautiful sunset, always keep going and don't let fear stop you.

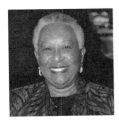

Vigilance

BY SONIA CHARLES

"I feel like I have a new life and I'm going to take full advantage of it." — William Green

In August 2001 when I was diagnosed with stage III intraductal carcinoma I had no idea what that meant. Although I suffered many of the effects of chemo, surgery and radiation, those were only potholes in my road to recovery.

My experience led my sister to write a book on how to have a voice when breast cancer is the diagnosis.

I strongly believe that if I can provide even one person with the courage, strength and perseverance to understand that the diagnosis of cancer is not the end of the road — it is only just the beginning of a new way to live — we can and will survive and thrive!

A word synonymous with surviving and thriving is vigilance — continuing our medical follow-ups and vigilance with renewed self-care. There is broader discussion and information available to millions who are surviving for more than 20 years after diagnosis and there is help to defeat our lingering fear. Only when we are no longer afraid do we begin to live.

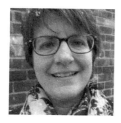

My Favorite Side Effect

BY DARLENE CUNNUP

"It is during our darkest moments that we must focus to see the light." — *Aristotle Onassis*

This journey began for me at the age of 44. I was a photographer who never thought I would be a part of the Pink Sisterhood but in May 2011 diagnosed with stage IIIa triple negative breast cancer, I joined the club.

Life happens in between medical appointments, not during them. I was determined that my life would NOT consist solely of treatments, doctors, side effects, and medication schedules. In the midst of finding out about the breast cancer and that I had to have surgery, I was preparing eight photo exhibits.

I decided as a photographer I should document my journey in photos so that the people around me would have more of an understanding of what it is like to live with cancer through my camera lens.

I have been positive from the start, but like any part of life, you cannot smile constantly without having a few sad moments too.

I embraced every minute of what I was going through and with the help of my camera and passion for photography I was able to carry on. Life is my favorite side effect.

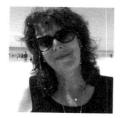

Paddles Up!

BY LINDA DALLMAN-REPP

"To advocate for yourself, you have to face those fears"

I received the devastating words on Friday, August 31, 2007. I never skipped my annual screening after my mom died of breast cancer at the age of 62. My first husband died of cancer in 2003. I had been remarried just a year when the news came. I was 57 years old.

A thousand questions raced through my mind. Do I tell my children? They were just getting over the death of their father. Both were finally getting on with facing their fears and living their academic dreams. This is what their dad wanted them to do.

They say adversity brings strength. This is true, I saw it with my late husband when he faced his terminal illness, I saw it with my current husband being orphaned at the age of eight and becoming successful on his own, and I felt it with my own cancer diagnosis. Face your fears.

Today, I am thrilled to be a team member of a dragon boat team. We are a group of strong women who have faced our fears and have all been bitten by the Dragon. Paddles Up!

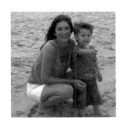

Rainbows after the Storms

BY ANGELA DUNCAN

"Never give up. FIGHT! We are warriors!"

In 2009, I was diagnosed with stage II triple negative invasive breast cancer when I was 29 years old. I was in a deep state of depression before my diagnosis but somehow the diagnosis made me want to fight back and live. I had a lumpectomy, chemo, and radiation. I felt like a caterpillar turning into a butterfly. Even though I was given a bad hand of cards, I made the choice to play them through and won.

Months later, I met my husband at a breast cancer awareness fundraiser. I also had a baby two years after the diagnosis. It's proof that there are beautiful rainbows after the storm. I had a recurrence in June of 2013 and had to have a bilateral mastectomy. It was hard, but again I was determined to face the challenges and become a stronger woman. In August, I found out I was pregnant again. We are now awaiting the birth of our second son, our second rainbow that appeared after the storm. It's hard to stay positive when you are given difficult challenges, but it's so worth it in the end. Never give up. FIGHT! We are warriors!

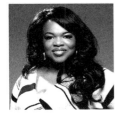

Divatude: Choose Beauty

BY DAPHNE EVANS

"Don't let cancer define you."

"We regret to tell you, but you have ovarian cancer." I've survived ovarian cancer (1998), breast cancer (2005) and spinal cancer (2009). At this time I am in remission. At my first diagnosis, I was shocked. I was in the best shape of my life: both my husband and I were body builders at the time in Florida. A hysterectomy at 35 and the idea of losing a major part of my womanhood plunged me into despair. My marriage dissolved and I moved to San Francisco. Even though I was still fighting, I became one of those career women overachievers.

In 2005, during a mammogram in preparation for a breast reduction, they found a "floater" in my left breast. I couldn't get past the hallway mirror, crying uncontrollably. I asked God, "Don't you think I've gone through enough?" But the next day I awoke with this peace of quiet resolve. One activity I always loved was going to spas. It was so wonderful that I went for an entire week! I decided I wasn't going to let cancer define me or allow it to rob me of feeling beautiful and creating joyous spa experiences for others.

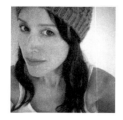

Note to My Past Self

BY MIYA GOODRICH-PHILLIPS

"Strength does not come from physical capacity. It comes from an indomitable will." — *Mahatma Gandhi*

Note to my past self...

It'll feel like your world's standing still. You will be breathless, lost, scared, helpless, and for a brief moment, you'll feel forgotten. The words, YOU HAVE CANCER will change you forever. The shock will soon wear off and things will begin to stabilize. You'll regain footing and you'll begin the process of rebuilding from the inside out.

You will never be the same. Cry for the person you're leaving behind and then try to let go. You may feel like giving up and that's okay. What you won't know is you're coming around a corner, so please hang on and keep pushing ahead. You'll feel alone, but holding your thoughts tight will only further isolate you. Let people in.

You'll cry hard over what you just accomplished and you'll watch in amazement as your body regenerates. You've had a rebirth of spirit, mind, and body. For the first time in your life you'll feel you are enough. You've seen the other side and found your way home. You have another chance. The future is unknown and unpredictable. Isn't it for everyone?

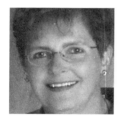

I Am Lucky

BY RITA KALKOWSKI

"Thirteen. Sound unlucky? Not to me."

My mother died of breast cancer in 1991 and my sister lost the same battle in 1993 at the age of only 47. I was always religious about my monthly self-exams, and while doing one 13 years ago, my life turned upside down.

At the age of 45, I stepped into the frightening world that included a biopsy, the VERY long wait for the diagnosis, a mastectomy, reconstruction, eight rounds of chemo, and six weeks of radiation. I had walked this path beside my family and friends before me, but it gets a lot more scary when you are the one lacing up the shoes. A low spot was landing in the ICU for five days with a blood clot by my port. But that's when I knew, that I was going to do everything to beat the odds.

After the Tamoxifen and Arimidex regimen, I thought I was on a smoother path. But then I had a heart attack and the detour included five stents. Now, 13 years later, I'm healthy, I exercise when I can, I'm positive, I won a Thrivers Cruise and I feel VERY lucky indeed.

Every Case is Different

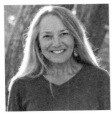

BY STASIA KERKMANS

"With the new day comes new strength and new thoughts."
— *Eleanor Roosevelt*

As a Physician Assistant in rural New Mexico I felt a responsibility for detecting breast disease in others but never dreamed it would happen to me. At 38 years old, I found a lump and went through mastectomy and chemotherapy when my twin daughters were only five years old. The fear of not surviving to care for them was the worst part of having breast cancer. After five years of tamoxifen I went through the trepidation of stopping treatment and a year later I found lymph nodes in my neck.

Since then I have had metastasis in bone, liver and lung, and each time through radiation, ablation and chemotherapy the cancer has abated. In fact my liver cancer is now undetectable!

Now retired from medicine, I meditate, do yoga, read, sing, attend support groups and am mom for my twins who are now 16. I've learned to no longer search for survival statistics, because every case is different and new treatments are developing all the time. You can learn so much from other patients who know what it is to live with cancer. They and my family inspire me!

Hang Tough! BY SUE KUEBLER

"You gain strength, courage and confidence by each experience in which you really stop to look fear in the face. You are able to say to yourslef, I have lived through this horror. I can take the next thing that comes along"
— *Eleanor Roosevelt*

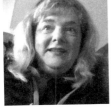

I will never forget how upset I was when I heard the news.

I'm very close to my Mom, and I told her immediately. Our friend Rose Kirby called me and told me that she had breast cancer over 30 years and she is a survivor.

Her advise was to "hang tough!" You can do it! Rose is my role model, she has had many problems in her life and she always says, "hang tough!" through it all!

Courage

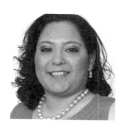

BY ROXANNE MARTINEZ

"I learned that courage was not the absence of fear, but the triumph over it." — Nelson Mandela

Courage is a word that often gets thrown around when you mention breast cancer. It may seem ironic for those newly diagnosed because we often feel scared and anything but brave. However, it takes an immense amount of courage to face a fear of the unknown.

My journey with breast cancer while pregnant taught me what it was to be courageous. While I was terrified for myself and my unborn child, I chose to fight breast cancer with hope and faith. I underwent surgery and chemotherapy while pregnant. There were days that I felt weak, both emotionally and physically. Still, I was fighting this battle for two and it required me to be brave. Despite a rough pregnancy and treatment, I delivered a healthy baby girl named Serenity.

Through breast cancer, I learned that courage doesn't always roar. Sometimes, simply living, holding onto faith and doing what we may be afraid to do takes courage. Fighting breast cancer often means doing whatever it takes to overcome the disease. Although we may not always feel strong, we face the pain, grief and loss associated with breast cancer head on. That, my friend, is courage.

The Stone

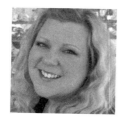

BY KARI MOROZ

"You can do this."

The leader of our spiritual retreat told us to each grab a small white stone out of a basket. Then she read Revelation 2:17 from a Bible.

"And I will give to each one a white stone, and on the stone will be engraved a new name that no one understands except the one who receives it."

Mine said "Courage." I scoffed. At the time, If I'd have chosen, it probably would have said "Average."

The next 10 years was a whirlwind of three corporate layoffs, Stage III breast cancer at age 29 with a newborn and a three year old, a horrific vehicle accident, and the leap of faith we took to start our own IT business. Before every major event, even though I'd tried to lose it, that stone would show up in the strangest places. Once I found it in a drawer and bawled uncontrollably, fearing it was a terrible omen. But over the years, it became encouragement somehow.. "You can do this"

Recently I found that stone, but instead of panicking, I laughed and said out loud "Bring it." Through the trials, God grew me into my name. I was meant for more than average. I became Courage.

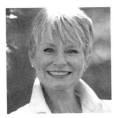

No More Dragons

BY JUDY PEARSON

"I learned that courage was not the absence of fear, but the triumph over it. The brave man is not he who does not feel afraid, but he who conquers that fear." — Nelson Mandela

Once upon a time all the smartest people in the world thought the earth was flat. Since they weren't sure of what might exist in the oceans, they took a better-safe-than-sorry approach and told everyone they were filled with monstrous dragons.

We assume what we don't know or don't understand will hurt us. That's certainly never more true than with a cancer diagnosis.

I was overwhelmed by the websites about my diagnosis (triple negative breast cancer), chemotherapy and reconstruction. None of the words were comforting. None of the photos calmed me.

When we're faced with challenges, the outcomes of which we're uncertain, our ancient brains instinctively steer us toward fear. But it doesn't have to be that way. Remember this joke: How do you eat an elephant? Answer: One bite at a time. As a joke, it's pretty cheesey. But as an ideology it's pretty good.

We can make our goals small, focusing on just 24 hours at a time. Research just one element of the challenge you face. Find one uplifting story of someone in a similar situation.

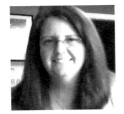

I Got Busy

BY CONNIE HOLLINGSWORTH SAUNDERS

"Failure is not an option."

I was 14 when I saw Mama in the hospital after her total mastectomy. I was a selfish teenager and my words were neither kind nor encouraging. I was scared.

Instead of getting down, I got busy! Mama had a thriving cosmetic business and I spent the next several months calling each customer to tell them the news and take their orders. The business experience I gained in those few months catapulted me to success. I gained a sense of confidence, a can-do attitude, and a real commitment to the goal of "failure is not an option."

Years later, a 30 year old close friend, Deneen, passed away from breast cancer and at her service they requested donations instead of flowers. I decided to get busy and dedicated a division of my cruise company to help raise funds for breast cancer.

Praise God, because of early detection, Mama is still here! 35 years cancer free! Today we laugh about what I said that day at the hospital.

People react to crisis differently. Words may not always be right, but actions speak louder than words. Get busy!

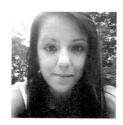

The Quiet Voice

BY LINDSEY SHELTON

My mom always quotes this when I'm having a tough day: "Courage does not always roar, sometimes courage is the quiet voice at the end of the day saying I will try again tomorrow."

I'm 22 and I live in a small town in Virginia. I just graduated from college in May 2013. The following September I found a tumor bigger than a bar of soap in my left breast. A core biopsy showed a spindle cell neoplasm. I had a lumpectomy to remove it. Pathology came back as an aggresive high-grade malignant phyllodes tumor (cystosarcoma phyllodes).

A second surgery was done to get wide clear margins which is necessary for a PT. PTs are very rare and it's even rarer for one to be malignant. It's not your typical breast cancer. In January of 2014, I had a left breast mastectomy and the beginning of reconstruction. Little is known about PTs and the reoccurrence rate.

My family, friends, and community are part of the source of my strength and I owe the rest to myself and God. They have pushed me forward to keep fighting an everyday battle.

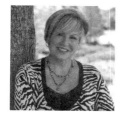

If I Could Go Back In Time

BY PEGGIE D. SHERRY

"It is all about your attitude."

It is much easier to be 10+ years out from breast cancer and take a gentle look back at the events that occurred during my cancer fight. Now, I wish it was possible to go back in time and tell my younger, terrified self "Peggie, everything is going to be alright."

My older wiser self would tell her that it was okay to cry and to calm her nerves when mammograms, tests, scans and blood work come back with frightening results. I would hug her and tell her that a medical team was going to fight to keep her safe and do everything they can to get her healthy again. She knows but needs reminding that friends will rally to help and comfort her.

Most importantly — it is all about your attitude. If you think you can kick it, your outcome is going to be a lot better than if you believe it will kick you. Finally I would hug her tight and tell her that her world will open up and that she would belong to a sisterhood of the most amazing courageous ladies in the world all answering to the word survivor.

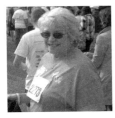

Cancer Doesn't Have Me

BY MARY T. SULLIVAN

"Meet everyone with kindness and compassion."

When I first thought about writing this article, I hesitated. I had been recently diagnosed with a reoccurrence of stage IV breast cancer that had spread to my bones and spine. I had been cancer-free for 10 years so the fact that it was back hit me like a ton of bricks. I had a mastectomy and chemotherapy in 2003 and after faithfully taking my preventative medication for 10 years, thought I had kicked cancer.

Treatment this time has been radiation, oral medication and monthly infusions of what is referred to as "bone glue." With the excellent care of my oncologist and tons of prayers and well-wishes from friends and family, I am feeling wonderful again. I think a positive, spiritual outlook contributes greatly to healing. I pray daily and try to treat everyone I meet with kindness and compassion.

I don't know how long God has given me, but the last PET scan looked great with only a minimal amount of cancer still there. I plan on being here for a long time to come, but still try to live each day to the fullest. My husband John remains the love of my life and my rock through this journey. I may have cancer again, but it doesn't have me.

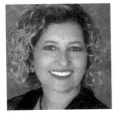

Be Your Own Advocate

BY VICKI TASHMAN

"Don't be afraid to ask important questions!"

I am a 10 year breast cancer survivor. When I was diagnosed, I assumed that my doctors would tell me what my treatment would be. Every time I left the doctor's office, I still felt in limbo about what to do and what not to do. They would give me options but never tell me "this is what you need to do." They would give me the statistics on each option, but I had to make my own decisions. I had to think long and hard about what my body was telling me, what was my intuition and what my husband's feelings were.

My lesson from this is to be your own advocate. Talk to the doc, talk to the nurse, talk to other survivors and do some research on the internet. Get educated and know what your pathology report means. What are the pros and cons of each treatment? If you have to have chemo, is it better before surgery or after? Get a second opinion and maybe even a third. You may need a second opinion on the pathology as well. Don't be afraid to ask some important questions! This is your body after all!

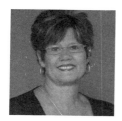

Everything Will Be Okay

BY KATHY VOYLES

"Trust your journey."

I was diagnosed in 2004 with breast cancer at the age of 41. I was so terrified because my mother passed away from ovarian and breast cancer in 1991. When I heard those words, "You have cancer" all I could think of was how my mother went through five years of hell. Two weeks later I arrived for my first chemo treatment, when I saw all those chairs with women hooked up to IV's I started crying hysterically.

I looked up and noticed an elderly woman walking toward my chair with her IV pole in her hand and in a sweet voice said, "Don't cry honey, everything will be okay." She continued to talk to me and I thought she is not that sick, I just might live through this and the next thing I knew my treatment was finished.

I can remember her last words to me were, "Trust your journey" and those are the words that brought me through my fight with cancer. I later found out that she was in a group of ladies that called themselves Stage 5 and Staying Alive. What a true inspiration she was in my battle against cancer.

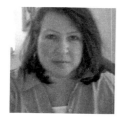

Welcome to the Pink Side

BY SHERRY WHEELER

"Experience it, every moment, good or bad, happy or sad, every precious moment."

When you hear the doctor tell you that you have cancer, it's like your whole world stops and you are frozen in that one horrible moment. You feel like you will never be able to move past it.

Life goes on in spite of our best efforts, in spite of how we feel, in spite of our fears, in spite of our standing still.

The important thing is to be there when it happens, living it and experiencing it, every moment, good or bad, happy or sad, every precious moment. Welcome to the Pink Side.

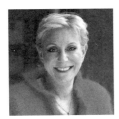

Choose Your Approach

BY MELANIE YOUNG

"Choose to be fabulous!"

Choice. This word is rich with significance with a cancer diagnosis. You may not have chosen to have breast cancer, but you can choose how to approach your treatment, nourish your mind and body, reduce stress, dress up or curl up, feel pity or pretty, and make the changes you choose take control of your life to stay healthy. Choose not to dwell on "why me" or "what did I do to myself to get cancer?" The blame game is tempting! I had a long list that I was convinced contributed to my diagnosis. Looking back may give you the insight and hindsight and foresight to change any negative lifestyle habits down the road, but how you approach cancer is your choice.

Now is the time to ask the right questions, get all the facts and work with your medical team to make smarter decisions to benefit you. Remember, having cancer does not mean you are contagious or untouchable. Having cancer is nothing to be ashamed about. Having cancer means that you need to be more pragmatic, have more patience and focus on turning a negative into a positive. Cancer may be bad, but you can choose to be fabulous.

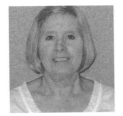

I Was Determined

BY VIRGINIA YOUNG

"When there is no struggle, there is no strength." — Oprah Winfrey

My husband Bart Young has been one of my biggest supporters. My sister had breast cancer in 1977; she's been cancer free for 37 years. At the time of her diagnosis, I remember thinking, 'I'll never get cancer,' but I did.

I'll never forget the day that I found out. I was on my way back to work when I received the call from my doctor. I cried so hard it hurt to drive. I called my husband and told him the news and again I cried so much I didn't know I had that many tears in me.

My sister was by my side, all the way from Kentucky to be with me before my surgery. She stayed the week with me following surgery.

I had radiation treatments every day for eight weeks. It was a long process and I remember having to take a nap at lunchtime, just to make it through the day. It was difficult and my strength was tested, but I was determined.

With the help of my family, friends and co-workers, I am proud to say that I have been cancer free for almost two years.

2013

Face *of* Inspiration: *Margo Johnson*

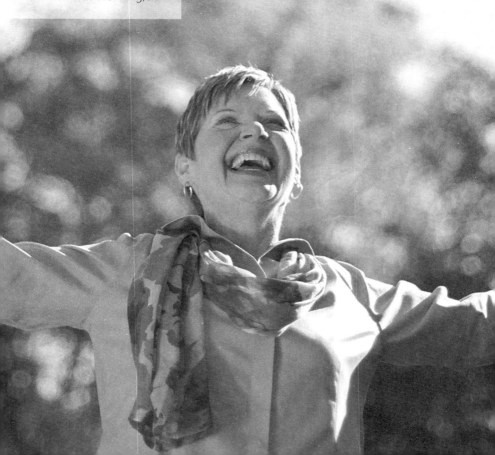

"Faith is
taking the first
step when
you don't see
the whole
staircase."
— Martin Luther King, Jr.

Steps of Faith

I grew up in central North Dakota with my parents and three brothers. After graduating from high school, I attended college and eventually became an RN. My loving husband and I have been together for over 30 years. We have two beautiful children and one adorable granddaughter.

My diagnosis was in March 2009 after a routine screening mammogram. I needed strength, hope and encouragement while facing the unknown. My inspirational words gave me a new perspective during my breast cancer journey. I reflected during those times of chemotherapy and for those moments following surgery.

It was a giant relief to discover that I only needed to take the first step. The whole staircase of tomorrow was not visible, but fear and anxiety were replaced by peace, joy and hope. I did not know what the future held, but I knew who held the future.

Now I look for opportunities to provide inspiration and hope. As a wife, mother, daughter, sister, friend, neighbor and nurse, I take advantage of opportunities to share words of encouragement to those in need. I take that step of faith each day and it transforms my entire outlook on life!

As a five year cancer survivor, I hope that this message of inspiration will motivate women to take action. Faith in God gives me confidence to do what I can today and keeps me from worrying about the future. The place to begin is by taking the first step. Each step I took built the confidence I needed for the next step.

As a winner of the ABC's Face of Inspiration contest, my life changed; the contest gave me the chance to be a voice of encouragement to other breast cancer survivors.

Get that mammogram because it could save your life! I did it and you can too. Live the life that God has given to you!

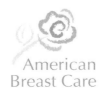

American
Breast Care

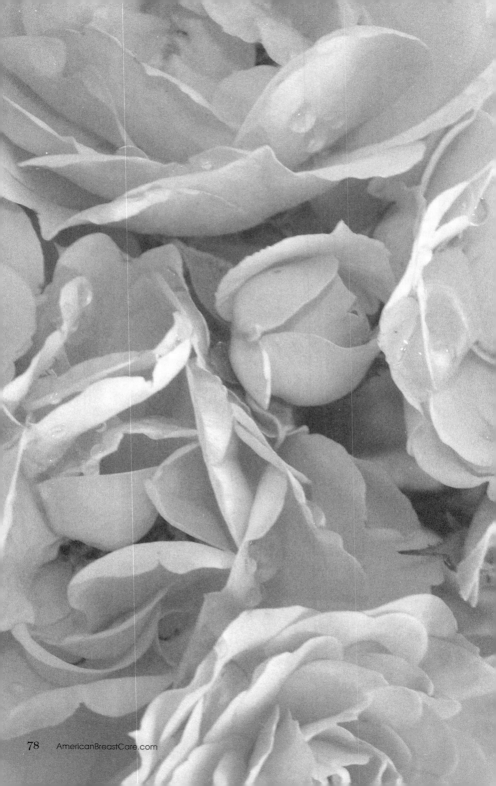

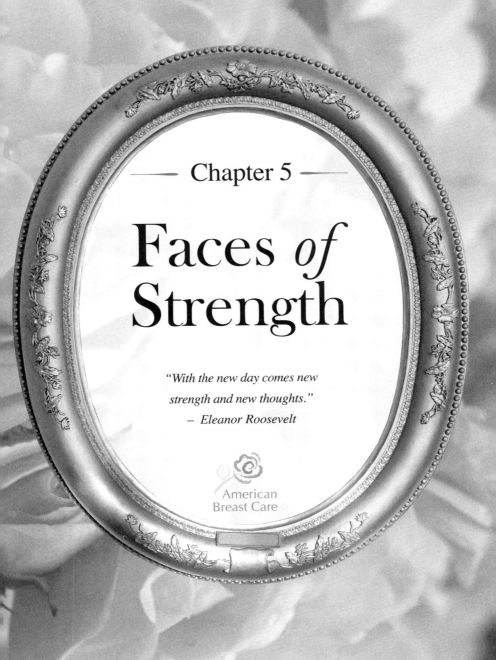

— Chapter 5 —

Faces *of* Strength

"With the new day comes new strength and new thoughts."
– Eleanor Roosevelt

American
Breast Care

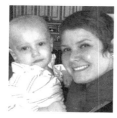

Imagine

BY AMANDA ADAMS

"Every adversity, every failure, every heartache carries with it the seed of an equal or greater benefit." — Napoleon Hill

Imagine being 32 with a three-month-old. You are getting ready for a wedding, which happens to be on your fifth year wedding anniversary, and then it happens. You feel it: a lump.

Imagine hearing the words, "I'm sorry, but it is cancer" on your third day back from maternity leave.

Imagine having breast cancer, stage II with lymph node involvement and BRCA 2+.

Imagine having a bilateral mastectomy, fertility, five months of chemo, losing your hair, six weeks of radiation and one year of additional targeted therapy.

Imagine this actually happening to you and imagine understanding why.

Imagine understanding it all happened as it did so that your child would not remember any of it.

Imagine understanding it all happened as it did so that your relatives could take precautionary action to save their lives.

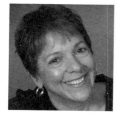

How Strong You Are

BY TAMI BOEHMER

A woman is like a tea bag; you never know how strong you are until you're in hot water. — Eleanor Roosevelt

Before I was diagnosed with metastatic disease, I remember telling someone going through it, "I don't know how you do it; I could never handle it." Now I know I can do more than handle it. It took a life-threatening disease to transform my life.

As Eleanor Roosevelt said, "A woman is like a tea bag; you never know how strong you are until you're in hot water." I believe my strength comes from knowing there is a Higher Power that loves me unconditionally and is guiding me to my highest good.

God is present when I make treatment decisions, leading me with that "gut feeling;" that still, small voice. God is present in all the wonderful people who have come into my life since being diagnosed with cancer.

My faith has been tested for sure. I've questioned God when scan results turned bad and when dear friends of mine have died. I don't believe God makes these things happen, but God certainly has helped me come out on the other side of these traumas.

I am grateful for all my gifts, most importantly my health, family and the amazing friends I've made in the cancer community. I am blessed.

It's time to live life like you did before you had breast surgery…

ABC®

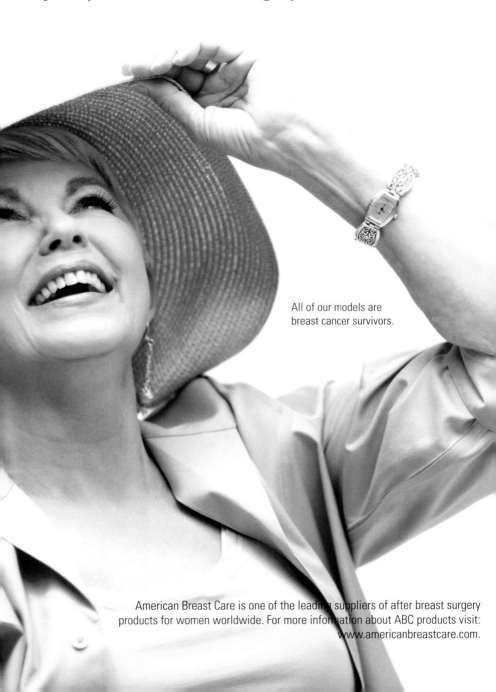

All of our models are breast cancer survivors.

American Breast Care is one of the leading suppliers of after breast surgery products for women worldwide. For more information about ABC products visit: www.americanbreastcare.com.

Everyday Bras

ABC features a collection of comfortable and easy to wear bras that remain undetectable under fitted clothing. Elizabeth is wearing ABC's Soft Shape T-Shirt Bra. This bra features seamless, molded foam cups with padded straps for extra cushion. It's the ideal bra for everyday wear.

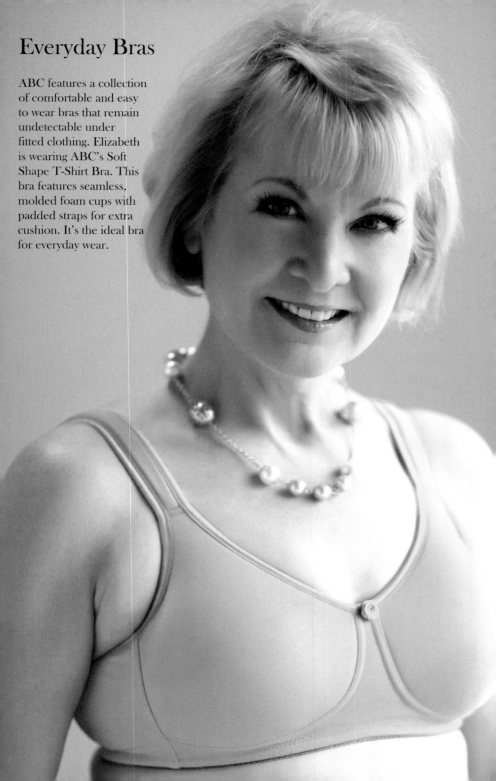

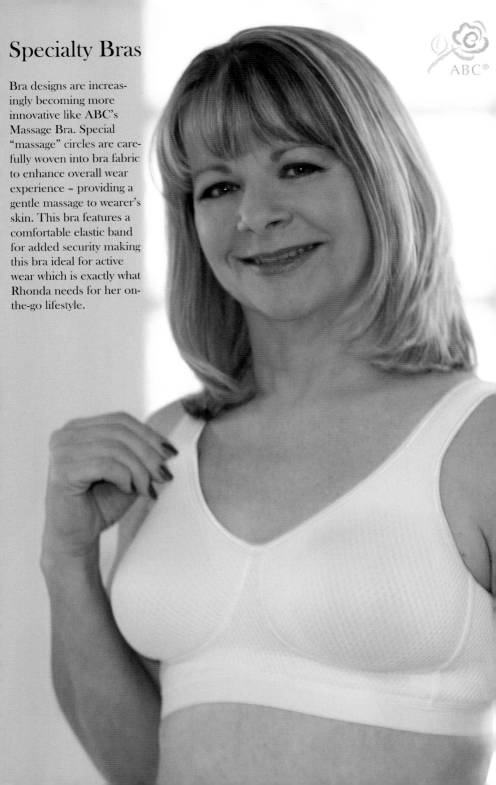

Specialty Bras

Bra designs are increasingly becoming more innovative like ABC's Massage Bra. Special "massage" circles are carefully woven into bra fabric to enhance overall wear experience – providing a gentle massage to wearer's skin. This bra features a comfortable elastic band for added security making this bra ideal for active wear which is exactly what Rhonda needs for her on-the-go lifestyle.

ABC®

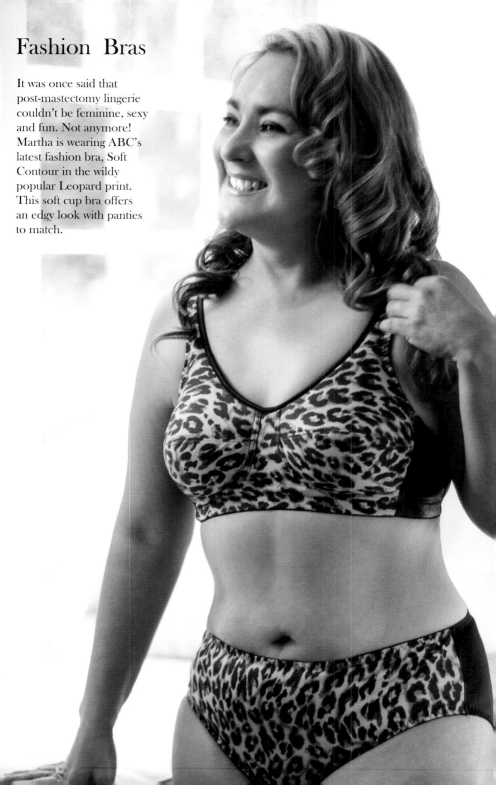

Fashion Bras

It was once said that post-mastectomy lingerie couldn't be feminine, sexy and fun. Not anymore! Martha is wearing ABC's latest fashion bra, Soft Contour in the wildy popular Leopard print. This soft cup bra offers an edgy look with panties to match.

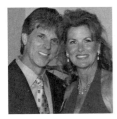

Thank You Mom

BY LYNNMARIE BOLTZE

"Find a way to help others."

Our story began in 1994 when my natural mother Mary Boltze was diagnosed with breast cancer and four other cancers. She was given three months to live with no options for chemo or radiation. She disagreed with the doctors and said "I will go when "I" am ready to go"; she gave us six wonderful months.

Her spirit, drive, determination, and fight to win were ***amazing***. I can't express in words the courage she showed all of us. Mom, I am proud of you and the battle you fought for yourself and all of us. Your strength and vigor impressed all the doctors and especially the family. I feel your vitality even today and know that your journey helped me to be the strong woman I am today.

While being her caregiver we were blessed to have many lengthy conversations about paying it forward. My promise to her was that I would find a way to reach and help others with cancer. I am proud to say that promise was fulfilled. To this day I have volunteered with Hospice and cancer nonprofits. Thank you Mom, for your inspiration and so much more!

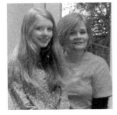

A Powerful Resolve

BY CASS BROWN CAPEL

"Your success and happiness lies in you. Resolve to keep happy and you shall form an invincible host against difficulties." — Helen Keller

While seeking fertility options, the doctor explained to me that it would cost between $20,000 to $30,000 for me to be able to increase my chances of conceiving a child. Too much of what he said made me think his way was like breeding an AKC puppy.

I walked out of there realizing that NOT having a child was NOT an option. All I could think was "I'll show him. Don't tell me I can't have a child!" My resolve was so powerful — it had to have been sent by God. I think whatever unconscious fear or ambivalence I'd been harboring was lifted at that moment.

I am now 60 years old. I was diagnosed when I was 32.

I have a lovely 14 year old daughter who is kind and decent. I've raised her with the same "never give up and never accept no" attitude which is how she talked me into getting her first horse.

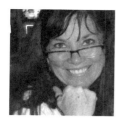

Never Doubt Your Strength

BY CHARLENE CATTOI

"You are a survivor!"

Never doubt the strength you don't even know you have!

And when you feel like you can't breathe... your body will take over and gasp for that breath.

Then take that deep breath! Feel it, then do it again!

I believe tears cleanse the soul! So no apologies. Go ahead and cry.

Because you can be happy, sad, grateful, scared — it doesn't matter!

We want control of our life to be what it was or what it we thought it was suppose to be. But what we have is here and now, and cancer sucks!

What we can control is how we handle what lies before us and that means moving forward one step at a time. Focus on the end of the journey and find the caregivers and the warriors who will walk with you giving support.

There will be times they are in front dragging, behind pushing, or even carrying us to help where needed!

You are a survivor! One day at a time!

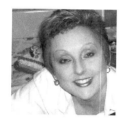

My Dad Walks With Me

BY KIMBERLY DAVIS

"The future belongs to those who believe in the beauty of their dreams."
— Eleanor Roosevelt

No one ever expects to be diagnosed with cancer. In October 2006, I was diagnosed with an advanced stage breast cancer. I was in disbelief and afraid that I wouldn't see my son reach his 7th birthday, or even reach my own 43rd birthday. From the very first doctor's appointment, I had strength from my family and friends. Mom helped with taking care of my son, Dad went with me to chemo treatments and friends wouldn't let me give up. I remember hearing my Dad cry one night at bedtime and I realized how hard my diagnosis was on my parents. My Dad never cried — he was a retired Army soldier — proud to wear the uniform and serve his country. Little did we know that Dad was very sick. On February 26, 2007, four months to the date of my diagnosis, my Dad was diagnosed with multiple myeloma. Now we both were patients at the same cancer center and even shared the same doctors. Despite a courageous battle, we lost Dad on August 1, 2011. To this day, I am cancer free and continue to make those visits to the oncologist, knowing that my dad is always walking with me.

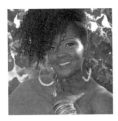

A Touching Journey

BY REVEREND TAM DENYSE

"The King will replay, "Truly I tell you, whatever you did for one of the least of these brothers and sisters of mine, you did for me."
— Matthew 25:40

Touch, quite possibly the most soothing thing we will ever know as a human is a warm touch. As a young girl, I watched my mother Carrie endure domestic abuse. Despite this horrific experience, she always found the will and the time to give back to others through community outreach. Sadly, her abuser took her life when I was 11.

Less than a month ago, I buried my son. I will miss his touch but will carry him in my heart forever.

Personal loss and pain has led me to give to others. When I was diagnosed with stage IIb breast cancer in December of 2004, I decided to be the voice for the silence that plagues the African-American community. We need to talk about the ills which plague us and seek resolution. Throughout treatment God was my foundation and He continues to be my driving force in my advocacy and outreach.

I founded an organization to show survivors that despite cancer, they can live life to the fullest. My imprint on the world will be a legacy of courage, faith and strength. Your faith must be stronger than any harm which may come your way.

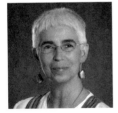

Stand a Little Taller

BY JANET FALON

"What doesn't kill you makes you stronger." — Sung by Kelly Clarkson

For five years I've taught journaling and expressive writing to people with cancer. One day I used the then-recently released song by Kelly Clarkson, "What Doesn't Kill You Makes You Stronger," as a writing trigger, and asked them to write how having cancer has made them stronger.

." . . what doesn't kill you makes you stronger, stand a little taller . . . what doesn't kill you makes a fighter . . . "

Participants were invited to share their responses. "Having cancer has made me re-commit to my faith, which has made me stronger," one person replied.

"I've learned that I can live with more physical discomfort than I thought possible," said someone else.

One woman cried as she said, "I'm so much stronger than before I had cancer. I now know I can live with being extremely anxious and go about my business."

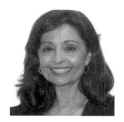

Grateful for Every Moment

BY ERIKA LANDAU FRAENKEL

"Healthy mind in a healthy body."

I am a pediatrician. I scheduled my first mammogram after finding a lump in my breast. It was negative but the radiologist ordered an ultrasound. The phone rang while I was seeing one of my babies. I picked up and heard "I am sorry but the lesion is malignant." I could not react or say anything. I continued the visit with the mom and her baby. The rest is somewhat a blur. I had a lumpectomy and radiation.

The lack of rest took a toll on me. I experienced pneumonitis, intense pain from the scar, fasciitis, fatigue and depression. I did not tell anyone about the cancer except my close family and a few co-workers.

Ten years later, I am grateful for every moment I have. Think positive and do not be shy in expressing your feelings. It is okay to be scared, it is not a sign of weakness. Do not go through this alone, allow people to help. Eat well, exercise, dance and have fun. Look well even during chemo. Use fun wigs and put on makeup and crazy jewelry. Cherish every moment you have.

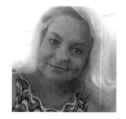

Being True to Me

BY HEATHER INGO-NUTILE

"I have cancer but cancer doesn't have me."

I was 32 years old, stage IIIb breast cancer of the most aggressive kind. It was 2004.

The word aggressive was used over and over again as well as conversations of odds of survival. In my head the only words I heard were "I will survive, I will do it my way." So I began my fight like a girl in lipstick and heels.

I had chemotherapy, a mastectomy with a staph infection in the middle. Reoccurrence wasn't a fear but it quickly became reality; however survival was still the only option. My goal was seeing my daughter's 18th birthday and sharing all the amazing moments in between. I knew if I kept running especially in lipstick and heels I would survive.

There have been good days and plenty of bad but they have been honest days of living life the best I could and being true to me. I have cancer but cancer doesn't have me. In March 2014, I celebrated 10 years of surviving what they thought I couldn't. Next year my daughter turns 18. I will never stop running or fighting in my lipstick and heels which means I should probably buy more shoes.

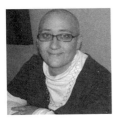

I Finally "Got It"

BY SHELLY JONES

"Persevere."

I was diagnosed with advanced breast cancer in 2010 when I was 35. I was a mom to three young children, and it was my daughter's birthday.

But I persevered. After eight crazy months, I began to search my soul for answers. "What did I ever do to deserve this hell? Why me? How will I ever be the same again? Why didn't anyone ever tell me "you are not untouchable... cancer can find you?"

Eventually I 'got it.' This horrendous thing happened for a reason. To go through it and come back stronger. To show others "I did it." To inspire women from all ages, races and all walks of life to be aware. Without going through breast cancer, I never would have been able to inspire the women in my life.

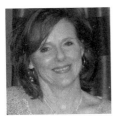

Together

BY CINDY LANE

"You never know how strong you are until being strong is the only choice you have." – Bob Marley

It was a beautiful summer day and I was having back pain again. I saw my internist and he ordered a CT scan of my pelvis and spine. Over kill I thought, but I was a good patient and went for the scan. I took a peek at my scan on their computer. I said to myself, "Oh my God, it looks like cancer." More tests, two biopsies, and three weeks later, it was confirmed that my breast cancer from 14 years ago was back now in my bones.

I fought this battle and won before, I can do it again! Then I learned what really was going on. Not only was the cancer back but I was told it was incurable this time. My medican team could only treat my symptoms. This was going to be a different battle.

My family and friends have rallied around me. We are traveling this unknown journey together. We've had some crazy times that made us laugh until we cried. Yes, I've had rough days, but I know I will also have wonderful ones to look forward to.

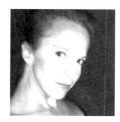

Live Legendary

BY TRACEY LANG

"Find joy and NEVER settle."

Not a single one of us picks cancer, why would we? This thing that has decided to take up residence in our bodies robs us of so much.

But I am inspired by the many people I know because of this disease and I thank them for being unique. Each had a special message:

Jennie used her attitude to grrrrrr her way through life. Nancy W reminded me that, "There is no try. There is do or do not." Dayna V pointed out that if you were an a — hole before cancer, you're an a — hole after cancer." Courtney C said, "It can take away my freedom, but it can never take my air guitar!" Jen S taught me to "live legendary." Jen E said, "Cancer lives with me. I do not live with cancer. Laura R.G. made me laugh. Lisa C started the flat person on a stick craze. Mary C told me that I can choose to dance in the rain.

I am thankful for my amazing friends that this c thing brought into my life.

Live. Love. Laugh. Smile. Be happy. Find joy and NEVER settle.

I never have. BACI

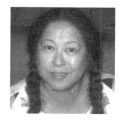

Aloha

BY LUHUA PETTAY

"May love, respect, and trust flow from me to you and from you, return to me."

I believe we are all spiritually unique and beautiful and that we need to believe in ourselves and in our true self. Love your self unconditionally. I did and still do and I made it, so why not you? There is so much positive power in perseverance and patience. Participate in guided meditation groups, gentle yoga, and consume only nutritious unprocessed food. Defeat the cancer; don't allow it to dominate your life. Communicate with your heart, not your mind which is too cluttered up with confusion and excuses that get in your way. Remember that fear is a choice and you don't need it, so it's best not to accept it into your life. Aloha means to embrace the life force within your earthly form. I am Hawaiian and I choose to share the spirit of aloha.

Aloha is:

Kindness expressed with tenderness

Unity expressed with harmony

Agreeableness expressed with pleasantness

Humility expressed with modesty

Patience expressed with perseverance

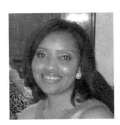

You're Strong

BY KERRI LOCKHART

"Beyond a wholesome discipline, be gentle with yourself. You are a child of the universe no less than the trees and the stars... And whether or not it is clear to you, no doubt the universe is unfolding as it should." – Max Ehrmann

I still remember the fear that followed the words "you have breast cancer." I remember feeling completely overwhelmed and all I wanted was for my life to go back to normal again. I also remember feeling so alone—like no one understood what I was going through. I was so relieved to learn that my feelings were completely normal. I was even more relieved to meet many wonderful women who have done this before me and understood firsthand what I was going through.

If you're feeling fearful, angry, and uncertain or a host of other emotions, I encourage you to connect with a survivor. Having other women with whom I could process my feelings, along with seeing survivors on the other side of the diagnosis really gave me hope.

Remember that you're strong and there is a sorority of survivors cheering you on every step of the way. May God bless you on this difficult but very important journey.

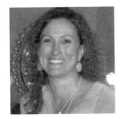

Life to the Fullest

BY JENNIFER MAGNANT

"It's only when we truly know and understand that we have a limited time on earth and that we have no way of knowing when our time is up, we will then begin to live each day to the fullest, as if it was the only one we had." – Elisabeth Kubler-Ross

I was diagnosed with invasive breast cancer at age 37. I was in shock, I was angry, and all I could see was my children's lives without their mother. They were ages 5, 9, and 11 then and I will never forget the look of fear on their faces. I realized at that moment that I would live. I drew my strength and courage from them and began the journey.

My life's purpose and mission came to light. I would do anything I could to help others with a cancer diagnosis. Six years later I help lead events to raise money and to make a difference! I have also joined a special group to be a support person for those newly diagnosed. The emotional strength that I received — and that I give — is the reason that I now live life to the fullest... every day!

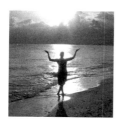

The Strength Within You

BY BEVERLY MCKEE

"The journey through breast cancer treatment is harder than we want it to be, but easier than we fear it to be. You have the strength within you to get through the dark days. You are a breast cancer warrior."

Being diagnosed with breast cancer is life changing. Everyone copes with breast cancer in their own way. I chose to view my breast cancer diagnosis as a storm. Storms blow into our lives and back out again, but even the biggest storm eventually runs out of rain.

There were dark days, but I searched for the rainbows through the storm every day. Now that my treatment is behind me, I look back at the many positives that came out of this journey. As unbelievable as it seems, breast cancer has changed my life for the better in countless ways. Given the choice, I would never have been diagnosed, but I would have missed out on the many amazing rainbows that were only observable in the midst of the storm.

Remember that it's okay to feel any and all emotions. My hope for you is that you will find the courage to search for your own rainbows through the storm.

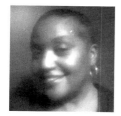

I Will Let My Light Shine

BY SHARAHN MONK

"Our deepest fear is that we are powerful beyond measure... As we let our own light shine, we unconsciously give other people permission to do the same."
— Marianne Williamson

I was preparing for my first round of six chemotherapy treatments and I was afraid. I didn't know what to expect. I needed to calm my thoughts so I began to pray. As I prayed, I looked out the window to see a beautiful blue sky with a brilliant sun displaying her rays upon the deep green of the earth's landscape. In that moment, I felt that day was created just for me and the journey was about creating my own atmosphere (my attitude) and what I chose to focus on. The fight for life was not only physical but it was also mental, emotional and spiritual.

To move forward, setting my attitude was my daily intention. Through the healing journey, I grew in strength and faith. Just as the earth's landscape is meticulously designed, so am I. I am a whole woman. Hair and breasts do not define me. Like the rays from the sun, my true self emerges — embracing my new perspective. Because I have life, I will let my light shine.

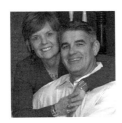

The Best is Yet to Come

BY TODD AND BECKY OUTCALT

"Celebrate the help you receive from others."

Twelve years after a breast cancer diagnosis and treatment, we are still married and life has been good. Although cancer itself is never welcomed, it has changed our lives in a myriad of ways. Like many women who survive breast cancer, Becky switched careers—returning to school to become a middle school science teacher and now a principal. And Todd has helped many men help their wives through breast cancer.

What have we learned through this experience? First, there is life after breast cancer—and much to look forward to. Our daughter is now married and our son is in college. We learned that we had many good friends, people who were willing to help. There are many caring people. Although it has always been more difficult for us to receive (we love to give), we had to learn how to accept help from others and, in fact, celebrate it.

And now, looking back, we can honestly say that the best is yet to come. Being a breast cancer survivor (and a caregiver) is more than just survival. It is an opportunity now to help others on their cancer journeys. After all, we've been there. And we all have more to learn.

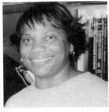

Living Life Fully

BY KIMBERLY PARKER

"You may encounter many defeats, but you must not be defeated. In fact, it may be necessary to encounter the defeats, so you can know who you are, what you can rise from, how you can still come out of it." — Maya Angelou

In August 2009 I was diagnosed with two forms of breast cancer. I used writing as a form of therapy to help me through the process. Writing was again beneficial when I had to have a hysterectomy due to possible early stages of ovarian cancer.

Even though this alien form inside of my body was trying to break me down, it was the love and support of my family that helped me. My relationship with God continues to grow and I trust that God has my best interest while I go through the fog.

My strong will to declare cancer out of my body as an unwelcome guest empowers me to live each day of my life fully.

My experience as a former police officer and navy veteran has taught me great things about strength, fortitude and being resilient. It also helped me see that I enjoy being of service.

Living life fully means being with my family and friends and helping others.

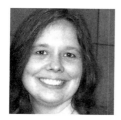

Support to Rejuvenate

BY MELISSA PASKVAN

"Find a new normal and live again."

In 2009 at age 41, I found my lump by chance when I felt something under my breast. My mammogram did NOT detect my 2cm tumor because of having dense breast tissues. It was thought to be just a cyst, but I insisted on a needle biopsy right then and there. Then I received the dreaded call from my doctor and was told I have breast cancer... I was numb. I was really scared of the uncertainty. Suddenly nothing else mattered, I couldn't see past "today." Can you imagine all the fear racing through my head?

I learned that I had a rare and aggressive form of cancer that doesn't respond to hormone therapy; it was triple negative breast cancer. I knew I was in for a long fight ahead of me and had to be strong and stay focused as I started treatments.

After treatment, I've struggled some and felt lost. As I tried to figure out my new "normal" and live again, I turned to a local cancer wellness center's group therapy for support that helped me rejuvenate my self-image and ease the transition that I've gone through.

As a four year TNBC survivor, I live life TODAY!

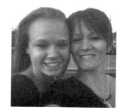

Strength Lives On

BY DEBBI RANDALL

"A grandma's heart is a patchwork of love" — Author Unknown

In 1958 I first heard the words breast cancer and they were only said behind closed doors. My grandmother had been diagnosed with breast cancer. She was 58 years old.

In 2001 I heard those very same words. I had breast cancer. I was 51 years old.

I remember my grandmother, a farmer's wife who lived in a house without an inside toilet or running water, always smiling thru the pain and the depression and never giving up. I can still see her sweeping her kitchen floor. She had the broom in her one good hand (that wasn't still bandaged) and the dustpan in between her toes. There was little that was done back in the 60's. My grandmother lived to be 87 years old.

I think of her while I am fighting this disease. I am now on my fourth recurrence. Family and friends are a big part of my every day recovery. And the moments I don't think that I can continue, I have wonderful memories of the strength and resiliency of my grandmother.

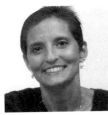

Just Reach Out

BY JENNIFER ROPER

"I can do this."

God has given me wonderful blessings, my loving husband, two boys and family. They mean the world to me and there is nothing that I wouldn't do for them. God has also given me and my family challenges to work through. Stage IV was my first diagnosis at age 31. The meaning of these words were completely devastating at first. It was the hardest thing I have faced. I did a lot of thinking, talking, praying and crying. Only then did the realization come to me. Hey, wait a minute I CAN DO THIS.

I'm strong, ready to fight and can show myself, my boys, family and friends that I'm here to stay and willing to do what it takes. It has not always been a walk in the park and I have gone through many obstacles but I keep fighting and working my way through them and I have no intention of giving up. This has taught me that life is worth fighting for through the good and the bad. Love, Hope, Faith and Prayers are always waiting for you, if you're willing to just reach out.

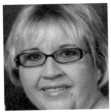

Strong I Am

BY SHARON SANEK

"You never know how strong you are until being strong is the only choice you have." — Cayla Mills

I was diagnosed with breast cancer on December 22, 2008. I had a left breast mastectomy and was HER2 negative. I did not realize how much I missed my left breast until I had my reconstruction. I am so amazed on how I feel about myself.

People say how strong and how proud they are of me; this makes me cry. It makes me stop and think of how strong we really all are. What breast cancer has taught me about myself and how God has trusted in me has been amazing.

I truly believe that God wants us to help others who are going through breast cancer and this is what I will always do. I have been blessed throughout my journey and

I want to inspire others because the women I have met have been such an inspiration to me.

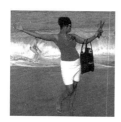

My Life Matters

BY DARLENE SHORTER

"The only courage that matters is the kind that gets you from one moment to the next." — *Mignon McLaughlin*

My world changed in October 2003 when my father called to tell me that my mom was diagnosed with parotid cancer. My heart dropped and I asked God why? Why? I was so afraid of her having to struggle and the thought of her being in pain was more than my heart could take. I was even prepared to take on her pain and diagnosis and even ask God to give it to me because I was younger and could handle it. I would have done anything for her.

Unbeknownst to me, that would become a reality four months later. I was diagnosed with stage III breast cancer. The same year that my mom was ill and it was not going to be an easy road for me. My oncologist explained the important details of my treatment. I asked why such a long list of treatment and procedures, he looked me in the eyes and said, "You want to live don't you?"

Less than a week later I was in the hospital undergoing the first of many treatments.

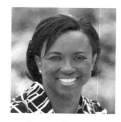

Live, Laugh, and Love

BY DAPHANIE BRANTLEY

"My great hope is to laugh as much as I cry; to get my work done and try to love somebody and have the courage to accept the love in return." — *Maya Angelou*

I was diagnosed with breast cancer at the age of 31. It was very devastating to me and my family. I can remember that day like it was yesterday and it changed my life forever. My sister was with me and I had an awesome doctor. My doctor was honest, and she put it to me; either I can beat this or it can beat me. Your choice! I chose to "live, laugh, and love life."

I knew then I wanted to live, but I gave myself two weeks of getting myself together mentally and spiritually. Also, I come from a loving, praying family and I had good family support. My grandmother gave me good wisdom — just listen to your doctor baby and you will be just fine with life. Because she was a survivor herself, she knew what it took to live a good prosperous life. She was diagnosed in her 40's and didn't die until the age of 95, from old age.

It was a six month process which included chemotherapy, radiation, and I lost my hair. I do not wish any of this on anyone, but I knew I wanted to live. I can say God is a healer, keeper, and he's awesome. Because I'm a survivor of 17 years, I can truly say that I have lived, laughed, and loved along this journey we call life.

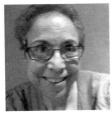

Blessed and Grateful

BY SHELLEY STEWART

"Hard times don't create heroes. It is the during the hard times when the hero within us is revealed." — Bob Riley

Oh the thoughts that encompass you when you first learn you are going to be a mom. The incredible joy and anticipation of the life you wish for your first-born. But, because kids don't come equipped with a user manual or a crystal ball to show you their future, you learn as you go. My first-born, Dana Anne Stewart, grew up to be an amazing, accomplished young woman. Independent, free-spirited, intelligent, kind, caring, just the kind of persona you would wish for if you could!

How the world changed on July 13, 2010. Dana, 32 years old, learned she had breast cancer. She picked herself up and plunged onto her road to treatment, recovery and LIFE! My husband and I helped when we could. She lived in Milwaukee, we were in suburban Chicago. But this girl did it all herself — doctor visits, mastectomy and reconstruction, and chemotherapy. She's back in Chicago now with a fabulous job, fabulous apartment, and fabulous friends. She is remarkable. She is healthy. I am a blessed and grateful mom!

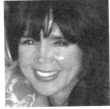

Becoming More

BY THERESA STEJSKAL

"Cancer is tough but I'm tougher."

I am 55 years old. I was diagnosed with breast cancer when I was 45.

As a woman in the prime of her life, the worst thing that could have happened to me was losing my breasts. It was my self-worth in life and validated by the universe. When my doctor called to give me the news, her words still ring in my head to this day. "I have good news and bad news. The bad news is... it's cancer. The good news is... we can take the breast." "Excuse me?" I sobbed... "What was the good news?" These were words I could have lived without ever hearing in my lifetime.

At that moment I felt like everything that made me a woman died and I wanted to die as well. Yes I know how stupid that sounds now, but at that time it was a very reasonable solution for me.

Today I celebrate being a strong woman and the acceptance of becoming more than my breasts. Now I can truly say I'm more than I've ever been.

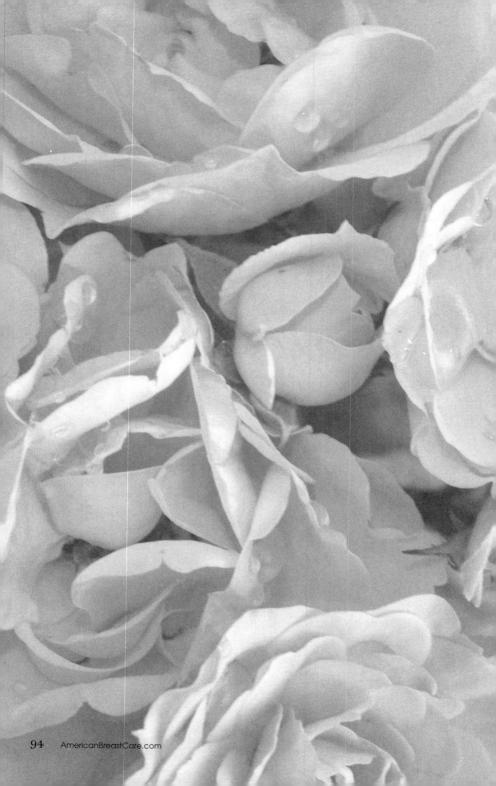

94 AmericanBreastCare.com

Chapter 6

Faces *of*
Inner Beauty

*"The beauty of a woman is not in the clothes she wears,
the figure that she carries, or the way she combs her hair.
The beauty of a woman is seen in her eyes, because that is
the doorway to her heart, the place where love resides.
True beauty in a woman is reflected in her soul. It's the
caring that she lovingly gives, the passion that she shows
and the beauty of a woman only grows with passing years."*
– *Audrey Hepburn*

American
Breast Care

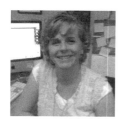

Embrace Love

BY ROBYN BROWN

"Your body will change but not your spirit."

If I could give a newly diagnosed woman some advice, it would be to embrace all the love that will surround you. I have met so many wonderful women who have gone through this experience. I feel like they are my sisters. We share stories, tears, and laughter. Breast cancer sucks but the people you will meet will change your life for the better. Your body will change but not your spirit. The woman inside doesn't change, let her shine through. I feel like I conquered a monster, the monster being the big "c." I never knew I had this much strength inside me, for this new found strength, I am grateful.

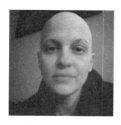

I'll Be Back

BY RACHEL BURNS

"The real glory is being knocked to your knees and then coming back. That's real glory." — *Vince Lombardi*

Today, the day before my last chemo, I find myself sick in bed, with just a few eyelashes, bald, losing fingernails, sensitive to almost all makeup, red nosed from using too many tissues. Really, the worst I have ever looked.

I took this photo after my last concert in October, a week before chemo started. I found myself upstairs alone at my mom's house; downstairs the house was filled with the laughter of friends and family. I knew in that instant that this was one of the last times in a good long while — if ever — I would look like this. The thought that I may not survive this battle, I may not live to see my hair once more or my youthful skin. I'm not one to spend a lot of time in the mirror, but I took the time, said goodbye to this lady and youth and I shed a few tears. I knew the journey would strip me of so much. It was a unique moment — I knew I wanted to keep it forever. The road is long, but I'll be back. I'll be different, but I'll be back.

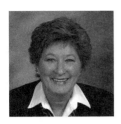

Take Time To Chuckle

BY MARY CATHERINE CARWILE

"Always laugh when you can, it's cheap medicine." — Lord Byron

Sometimes all it takes is a little humor. If I'm having a hard time in life, laughter always brings me back to myself and then I'm able to look at life again, renewed.

I became a flight attendant not too long after I had my mastectomy... at age 55, no less. I remember one day deplaning from a long trip. Waiting in the jet way was a dear friend, a classmate of mine from flight attendant training.

We ran up to each other and threw our arms around the others' shoulders. What happened next still makes me laugh. My friend, so delighted to see me, gave an extra umph to her hug. She squeezed me about shoulder blade height, right behind where my right breast used to be. Her arms around my back, my body was against her body and she placed it just right because the prosthetic inside my bra gave a loud and hearty burb! It was hilarious! She looked at me; I looked at her and the laughter grew until we were about to, well, you know. Nobody around us was the wiser and thought we were just happy to see each other.

Remember, we can find laughter almost anywhere.

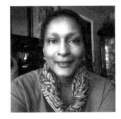

My Favorite Colors

BY HELENA DAVIS

"Fight the battle with all you have inside."

Before my journey with breast cancer, my two favorite color combinations were actually pink and purple. I had a small business and these were my theme colors.

I loved the way these two colors simply complimented each other. How ironic and little did I know that these two colors would be the theme colors of "my new normal."

Pink representing breast cancer and purple representing "surviving breast cancer." I can hold my head up high and say that I fought this battle with all that I have inside of me and I encourage anyone facing this battle to do the same.

Cancer may have taken a lot away from me but not my love for pink and purple after all they are my theme colors; they represent my new life!

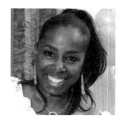

I Saw Only One Thing

BY JOANNE ENGLISH ROLLIESON

"The more challenging an experience, the greater the glory."

It gives me great joy to share my story! My struggle with cancer made me a stronger and better person, living life more abundantly. It has made a tremendous impact on my life and the lives of others because I share my story of survival, encouragement, and hope at every opportunity.

My story began at age 21 when diagnosed with stage IIIb Hodgkins Lymphoma. I had a new baby boy and much to live for. Although my parents were told I had only 6 months to live, I am now the proud grandmother of a 3 year old. Today, I enjoy good health and a vibrant life even after being diagnosed 30 years later with stage IIb breast cancer. Chemotherapy, radiation, loss of hair and appetite, doctors, medicines, and death staring me in the face AGAIN... I saw only one thing... LIFE. My mission now includes philanthropic, volunteer, and celebratory work for cancer organizations. I continue my professional career as CEO of a successful family-owned real estate company. As a two-time survivor, I thank God for sparing my life so I can make a difference in the lives of others.

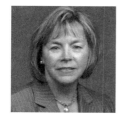

The Dance of Existence

BY JAN GROSSMANN

"Only 10 percent have the wisdom to accept both life and death as facts and simply enjoy the dance of existence." — John Heider, The Tao of Leadership

My breast biopsy brought shocking news! This couldn't possibly be correct! I ate right, exercised regularly, and had no family history of cancer. I was launched into a whirlwind of tests, uncertainty, terror, and unrelenting thoughts of life's end! Why?

The timing couldn't have been worse! Having resigned from my job a few months earlier, I was in the midst of a job hunt during a recession. I realized that if potential employers learned that I was undergoing cancer treatment, there would be no job offers. Therefore, I decided to share my news with only four friends, making the process of going through surgeries and radiation therapy extremely lonely and a somewhat surreal experience.

Cancer survival brings lingering fears. Honestly, though, the hardest challenge I've faced has been to deal with guilt — the guilt that I got better when others do not always get better! Why? But as John Heider suggests, I've learned to accept both life and death as facts and I've learned to simply enjoy the dance of existence! And what a wonderful existence it is!

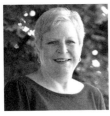

Be Glad You Did

BY BRENDA HAWKES

"The human race has one really effective weapon, and that is laughter." — Mark Twain

Hi, I am Brenda Hawkes. I was diagnosed in 2006 with stage III triple negative breast cancer. I found out soon after that I also have the BRAC 1 mutation.

Within six weeks I had lost my breast, my hair and my job. But I never lost my sense of humor. It was the humor that made the chemo, radiation, and nine surgeries tolerable. That is not to say, I was never angry... oh yes, I was angry. It was directed toward the lack of support that women get, the lack of compassion from employers, and the lack of understanding from people you just knew would be by your side completely.

It is interesting what I remember most is not the anger, but the humor I shared with my daughters, family and friends. We still laugh about the Razorback stickers on my bald head and the kitten I got for comfort which turned into the cat from hell. Humor is as important as any medicine available. Laughter just feels so good. And it is contagious. Even on your worst day share a smile, a laugh or even a giggle. Everyone will be glad you did.

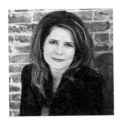

I Treasure Who I Meet

BY CHALENA HETZNECKER

"Kindness is difficult to give away because it keeps coming back." — Author unknown

Being a certified mastectomy fitter means that every day I meet ladies who are dealing with different stages of breast cancer.

Learning about their personal journeys in dealing with a breast cancer diagnosis is emotional and inspiring. Their quiet, gentle determination to beat cancer and to live their life to the fullest always makes me step back and re-evaluate my priorities.

They inspire me to treat each and every day as a gift and to realize the importance of everyone being kind and supportive to each other.

I hope one day my job will be obsolete and no one will have to go through having a mastectomy because this disease has been cured. Until then I will treasure getting to meet these amazingly strong women.

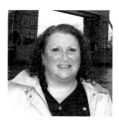

The Gift of Confidence

BY JILL FOER HIRSCH

"The goal is to live a full, productive life even with all that ambiguity. No matter what happens, whether the cancer never flares up again or whether you die, the important thing is that the days that you have had you will have lived." — *Gilda Radner*

I learned the lesson to appreciate life and not take too much for granted as a child; I was 9 years old when my father died at age 39. What he left behind are memories of a loving dad and a devoted husband and a man who made people laugh. He didn't live long but he lived well.

I could cower in fear and hope that nothing bad would ever happen to me, or I could embrace change; the good, the bad, even cancer, as part of life. Cancer gave me the gift of confidence. Knowing that I can handle whatever life brings gives me immense freedom. I'm not a victim of the past nor am I a prisoner of the future. I know how to live well and how to love well and I know how to make other people laugh in almost any circumstance. Nothing, and no one, can rob me of sense of humor and love of life.

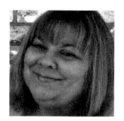

Heroes

BY VICKIE JENKINS

"Hero — A person noted for feats and courage and nobility of purpose."

When I was a little girl, I enjoyed reading comic books. I liked the colorful covers with the make-believe characters who were capable of saving the world.

Having a family history of breast cancer, I knew the importance of getting annual mammograms. At the age of 49, I was diagnosed with breast cancer. I went through a lumpectomy, brachy therapy (a form of radiation) and numerous doctors' visits. My personality changed from my usual happy self to someone that I didn't know. My simple life was turned upside-down. It was a rough battle, but I got through it!

Ten years later, the journey continues. With the help and support of family and friends, diet and exercise, annual mammograms and staying informed, it makes me stronger, living life to the fullest. I still think about heroes at times, not the make-believe characters but real people like myself and others.

I am a person noted for my feats and courage and nobility of purpose. I survive, I thrive and I am a hero!

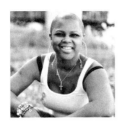

I Love Your Hair

BY SHEILA JOHNSON-GLOVER

"Embrace the new YOU."

"I love your hair." I get this all the time from women and men who have no idea the battle I'm currently fighting. Bald is beautiful. It's sexy, it's bold and it shows confidence. This is the first thing that I try to tell women when I talk to them about losing their hair while fighting cancer. Hair... it'll grow back. It does not define the person you are inside.

My name is Sheila Johnson-Glover and I'm bald. I was diagnosed December 2009 with stage IV HER2 metastatic breast cancer. Four years later, I'm still here — still receiving the healing power of Jesus and I'm still healthy. Did hair have anything to do with my healing? Nope.

Cancer will never silence my joy or steal my beauty. Cancer cannot take away the beauty that's already inside of me. Your hair will grow back and losing it is part of the process of beating cancer. God is so amazing and he has given me this journey for a reason. Embrace the new YOU. The new YOU is a Survivor. Did your hair have anything to do with that? Nope... so love your hair bald and all... I know I do.

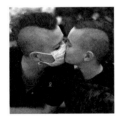

Who I Am

BY CARRIE ANN KEMP

"When you are at peace with yourself you shine!"

I stood in front of my full length mirror. Not a hair on my body from chemo. Both breasts taken by the surgeon. Drains hanging out of both sides. Scars and swelling from a complete hysterectomy. No make up. Not even pretty painted toes. My eyes sunken. I thought to myself... am I even a woman anymore? All of things that make me a woman are gone. What box do I check at the drivers license division? What am I now?

And it was in that beautiful painful moment that I realized what makes me a woman is on the inside. My heart. My soul. My spirit. How I love. That is what really makes a me woman. And when you are at peace with yourself you shine! And all of the things on the outside glow in wondrous beauty because of who you are on the inside.

I am a Mom. A daughter. A midwife. A healer. A teacher. A warrior. A winner. I am beautiful.

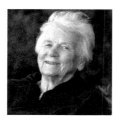

Do What Seems Right

BY JUDY KNOWLES (TWO TIME SURVIVOR BORN NOVEMBER 18, 1919)

"Do everything in moderation, even moderation."

Luckily my cancer was detected early — not past lymph glands, so no chemo or radiation. Two weeks past my first mastectomy my husband suffered a stroke, remaining on a feeding tube the rest of his life, April through August. Our 65th anniversary was June 9th, but how could it be celebrated? I spent the day with him as always then — at his bedside. I miss him very much. I thank God daily for our good memories, two special sons and their families.

After six years, the cancer returned. I wanted it out fast, but the surgeon was booked. So I traveled to help pass the weeks waiting. Once the pain pump was out, no additional medication was needed. My routine returned to walking two miles a day, volunteering with Hospice, Pregnancy Center and church events. In WWII, I volunteered in hospitals, the USO and 10 years at a nursing home. I found that volunteering diminishes personal problems. The past three years I've attended cancer weekends where each camper's story is unique, yet it's like we're in the same sorority. My advice is always do what seems right at the time and don't look back.

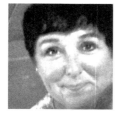

How You Live Your Life

BY SHARON KOGUTEK

"There are only two ways to live your life. One is though nothing is a miracle. The other is as though everything is a miracle."
— Albert Einstein

Sometimes it takes a crisis, an illness, a death of a loved one, an accident, a misfortune or a tragedy to turn your very secure, safe world upside down. Such was the case for me when I was diagnosed with breast cancer in October of 2003. After surviving chemo, radiation and eight different major surgeries as well as another cancer since that time, I view and dearly treasure the miracle of every day.

As Ralph Waldo Emerson said, "What lies behind us and what lies before us are but small matters compared to what lies *within* us." It's really what you do with your life and how you live it that matters the most. Sometimes it takes that crisis to shake you up and realize the beauty of everyday simple pleasure

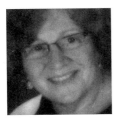

Your Love Needed

BY PAULINE LECLERC

"Live life better, not bitter."

I love the quote "Live, Love, Laugh"... and that is the way I took my diagnosis. I was 43 years old and had so much more living to do.

I seriously told the doctor: "Let's get this over with; I have my daughter's college graduation to attend! I do not plan on missing it." I often wonder how I really survived. But, in truth, my daughters were always there to support me... in person and in spirit. One of my best memories of this experience was when my nephew asked me to see my bald head. As I took off my bandana, the first words out of his mouth were "Boy, you look like Pepere!" (Pepere was my father.)

I continued to be positive each day, taking life one moment at a time. Through my experience with cancer, I learned to live outside my box and overcome many fears. Attending breast cancer retreats and breast cancer cruises have taught me that I am not alone on this journey. Someone out there always needs your story and your love.

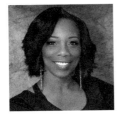

Living with Tenacity

BY ADRIAN B. MCCLENNEY

"Sometimes I sit and look at life from a different angle."
— Tupac Shakur

I was diagnosed with stage IIIb inflammatory breast cancer on May 19, 2011. That day transitioned me from a person who thought that being diagnosed with breast cancer was the worse day of my life into a better me.

I appreciate everything and everyone! I smile knowing that I am able to see the beautiful colors that the world has to offer. Watching the beautiful sky or the trees blowing shows me there is life everywhere. To hear rain drops or birds chirping are also sounds of life. I hope everyday we as people can live with confidence and tenacity. Use your courage to fight and push forward through challenges would be my words to the world. Never ever give up on life even if the situation looks impossible. I love being able to teach, advocate, inspire and motivate about breast cancer and that's very fulfilling to me. Remember to love, smile, and be happy just because you can.

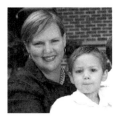

The Perspective I Now Have

BY LISA MILNE

"For I know the plans I have for you, declares the Lord, plans to prosper you and not harm you, plans to give you hope and a future."
— Jeremiah 29:11

I was diagnosed on October 1, 2008, the first day of breast cancer awareness month. I found the lump while showering. I thought because my cycle was starting, it was normal. My best friend is an ultrasound tech and I went to see her. I could tell by the look on her face it was not good news.

Since having cancer, I have had another child. He is now two years old. My boys and my husband are my inspiration. I thank God every day for them.

I take time to take care of myself. I enjoy life! I wish every person has the perspective that I have now. It makes life so much sweeter.

My greatest challenge was the fact that I was so young. I had no one my age that I could talk to about what I was going through. I did make a friend online who was diagnosed the same day as me and she was only a couple years older than me. She and I are still in touch.

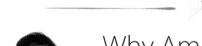

Why Am I Here?

BY GABBY MOTTERSHEAD

"Here is the test to find whether your mission on Earth is finished; if you're alive, it isn't." — Richard Bach

We were not born to worry and struggle, yet many women live in a constant state of stress, like I used to.

I had a difficult childhood, including abuse, abandonment and was placed in the care of the local authority at age 15 and pregnant. I had my baby for all the wrong reasons; I just wanted someone to love and someone to love me back. Aged 18 I met my husband. I worked hard, studied part time, and at age 39 was a director of a large company and graduated with my MBA. On the outside I looked like a successful woman. I had overcome my childhood; work gave me status.

At age 44, I was diagnosed with inflammatory breast cancer. I had chemotherapy, mastectomy and radiotherapy. I realized not only did I need to heal my body, but I also had to heal my soul and nurture my spirit. But I still asked why am I here?

I realized my life purpose and I now help other women to do the same.

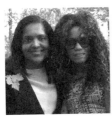

Dance Ballerina
For my sister and BFF, Pamela Michelle Garnett

BY LEPENA POWELL-REID

"Our roots say we're sisters, our hearts say we're friends."
— *Author Unknown*

With every new day, she does not give in
She gets up, Dresses up
With an award winning charm
A visit to her doctor does not always denote success,
She takes it as a blessing and steps over the mess.
She glides like the fair ballerina that still lives inside,
And remains open to the potential to live and to strive.
Her hard drive is wired to overcome this disease
She and her doggie both adorned in their pink,
Raising a paw and a hand to overcome the defeat.
A walk, a dance in the streets, a trophy of hope determined to win,
A vision she has as the tears may fall.
A universal strength. A strong sisterhood.
Survivors joined in a circle filled with love!

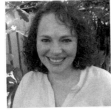

Counting My Blessings

BY NADINE ROSARIO

"The first wealth is health." — *Ralph Waldo Emerson*

Out of remission from invasive stage II triple negative breast cancer emerged the promise of a new beginning, a brighter tomorrow. The most challenging achievement of my lifetime inspired me to continue with my positive outlook, looking at what is and not what could have been.

The cancer I had was my greatest inspiration, teaching me to love myself by taking care of my health. The words "the first wealth is health," has provided me with words to live by. For example, I strive to educate and continue to take care of myself emotionally, physically and spiritually for the notable truth is that our health is the most important stepping stone in accomplishing anything. Being a part of something greater, such as my Heroines Choir Group, allows incredible healing through the power of singing. Comprised of victors and supporters of breast cancer, the choir provides great inspiration.

Learning to accept what I can control, acknowledging the things that are a greater challenge, leaves me triumphant in survivorship. Counting my blessings allows me gratefulness, for the sisterhood of all breast cancer survivors.

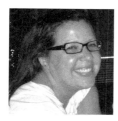

Living Everyday Life

BY DANA STEWART

"It's just words, not a state of being."

My defining cancer moment wasn't the diagnosis itself, but when it forced me to go back to my life. I chose to ignore the words "new normal." Why should I have a new normal when I am still me? I became a cancer survivor at the age of 32. It's just words, not a state of being. My first steps back into the real world after my bilateral mastectomy were less than glamorous. I could barely lift my arms and wasn't allowed to carry anything heavy. So, how was I supposed to take my cat to the vet? Desperate to be back to normal, I built a cat carrier out of a luggage cart and rolled my cat over to the vet myself. It was funny, but it was normal. I was not going to stop living my life.

From that experience to the next, and all in between, I learned a lot about myself.
I was of the mindset that cancer couldn't happen to me. It did.
I thought I couldn't survive cancer. I am.
I figured I would never get my life back. I have.
It's just now full of more crazy adventures, living the everyday life!

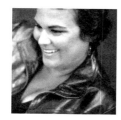

Parking is An Attitude

BY HAYLEY TOWNLEY

"Boobs may come, and boobs may go, but funny lasts forever."

When I recently went to have my hair done (I'm as blonde as I want to be!), it was threatening to rain. We all know what rain can do to salon-perfect hair.

I strolled into the salon and confidently told my hairdresser to give me bangs. This was a huge step for me.

I'll be honest. I might have asked him, "Would bangs make me look younger, or would they just make me look like I'm trying to look younger?"

Then I had a flashback to 2003. I won my fight against aggressive breast cancer at the age of 36. I was bald for a year. Honestly, what do I care if bangs aren't right for me? I know my hair will grow back.

I can change a lot of things in my life. Perspective is one of them.

My bangs look terrific (definitely younger!). I made it to the car with my salon-perfect hair. I survived breast cancer. And parking is an attitude.

Now go out there and make your own parking space in the universe!

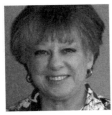

A Journey of Song and Love

BY DIANE VARNER

"I live as if each moment is my last and I trust God to lead the way."

I chose my journey to be one filled with joy and November 9, 2007 forever changed my perspective on life. A cancer diagnosis can be devastating and the treatment can be very difficult, but I vowed to make lemonade out of the lemons. With tremendous support of loved ones and friends, I have learned to play the hammered and mountain dulcimers, sang in a classic rock band, have seen the Passion Play in Germany, sang in the church Martin Luther founded in Worms, Germany, traveled to Costa Rica, and numerous other things I never thought I would do.

I now live as if each moment will be my last and trust God to lead the way, with music playing a very strong role in the healing process. Two years ago, I went back to work for a former employer and ironically, it is a mammogram facility. When a patient says to me "you have no idea how this feels", I can honestly respond, "I do." My life on this earth will end eventually, but until then, my journey will be one filled with song and joy!

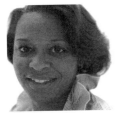

Keep Positive People Around You

BY CHARRON WALKER

"With God, all things are possible!"

I was diagnosed with breast cancer at the age of 32. My mother passed away from this disease at the age of 34. This experience has made me a better person. I would not want to experience that again, but it was priceless. I don't have to look at my scars and feel uncomfortable about my body anymore. My self-esteem has grown by leaps and bounds. I have learned from this experience that it does not matter who you are or what you've been through, you are beautiful in spite of your circumstances. Beauty comes from within and compliments who you are on the outside. It has also given a boost to my "I can do anything if I put my mind to it" attitude. The only roadblock is me and the limitations I set. Through this journey I found my purpose; I started a support program for young women survivors of breast cancer. I am able to tell breast cancer conquerors that your diagnosis is not a death sentence. I encourage all of you to speak life and walk in your destiny and healing. Keep positive people around you!

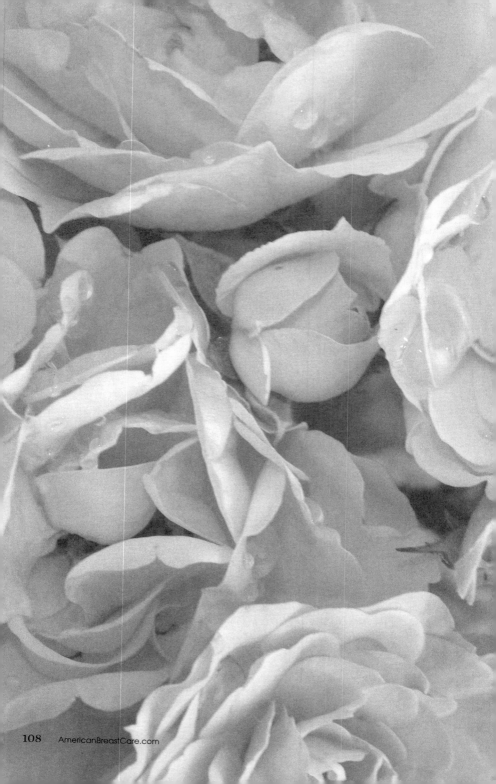

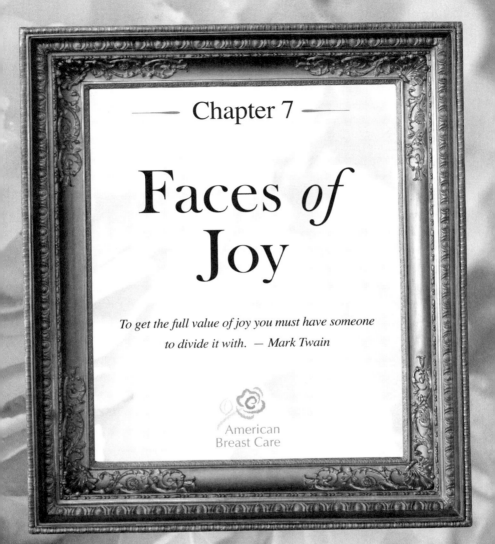

Chapter 7

Faces *of* Joy

To get the full value of joy you must have someone
to divide it with. — *Mark Twain*

American
Breast Care

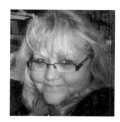

It's the Little Things

BY KAREN BELL

"Joy cannot be pursued. It is a state of being. It does not depend on circumstances, but triumphs over circumstances. It provides a gentleness of spirit and a magnetic personality." — *Billy Graham*

Leading up to the time I was diagnosed with breast cancer, my life wasn't exactly happy and joyful. In many ways, I was still grieving the loss of my daddy to cancer.

Oddly, breast cancer has brought me a deeper sense about joy and simplicity. I find that I pay more attention to the little things that we all take for granted, such as watching my grand kids play, the flowers that are blooming, and nature in all its beauty. It has put my life in order. I see things in a different light now. I thank God each and every day for healing me.

As I worry about my mother's aging health and well-being, I reflect how she brought joy and value to my life and to her grandchildren's and great grandchildren's lives. When I consider the little things in life that really aren't so little and the endurance and meaning that family provides, it truly adds up to joy.

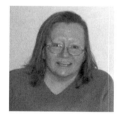

Soul Friends

BY EMILY TOWNSEND

"An old day passes, a new day arrives. The important thing is to make it meaningful." — *Dalai Lama*

I admit that I had taken my girlfriends for granted through the years. Most of our girlfriend group had gone our separate ways, sometimes exchanging Christmas and birthday cards. Once in awhile we would receive or send an email with a joke or a political assertion.

When I was diagnosed with breast cancer at the age of 58, I truly didn't know there was a deeper and more meaningful group of friends in the world. I learned from perfect strangers that there is a level of humanity that I had not experienced before. They had my back and I learned how to have their backs. You would think this is something I would have learned as a child, but nonetheless I am overjoyed to personally know women who help others to see beauty and meaning in life. If it took breast cancer for me to realize there is such a thing as soul friends, so be it. In the meantime, I am whooping it up with joy with my new friends.

Joyful to Help Others

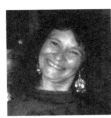

BY PAT HILL

"Normal is in the eye of the beholder." — *Whoopi Goldberg*

I am an nine year breast cancer survivor. Part of creating my new normal after breast cancer was finding joy in helping others who were facing breast cancer. My new normal also included being more thankful for family, friends and our small community that poured out their love. I am so thankful for the simple, yet beautiful things such as nature that I once took for granted. I am grateful my husband never left me and thankful how my eight year old granddaughter helped out as a caregiver. I now speak with others who are going through breast cancer and end up finding my best pink friends. Just as others reached out to me within my community, I want to help others.

At times, life is still challenging, but being thankful for the nine years the Lord has blessed me with makes a difference in how I face these hard times and being with family and friends brings me joy to get me through these hard times. I am fortunate in this new normal because I'm alive and life is beautiful.

Joy

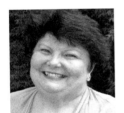

BY WENDY DOHERTY

"Joy is not in things; it is in us." — *Richard Wagner*

It took a breast cancer diagnosis and treatment to teach me the meaning of happiness and joy. From my perspective, the two are "joined at the hip."

Our options in life are:
- live with regret by looking in the rear view mirror of life
- live with angst by trying to see into the future
- live in the moment

The first two options are fear-based. We wouldn't think of driving our car by looking in the rear-view mirror. If we did, we would miss all the sights and sounds along the way. The same holds true for looking too far ahead. Select either option and we will miss the here and now.

If we choose to live in the moment, we will operate from a state of love. When we express this love by showing gratitude for whatever life has brought us at that moment, we can find our joy. We do not need perfect circumstances to have joy. It is within us. We only need to open our bag of courage to find it.

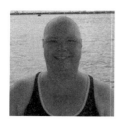

The Joys of Life

BY CRISTINE COSGRO

"A friend is a gift you give yourself." — *Robert Louis Stevenson*

I cannot talk about my experience with cancer, either as a stage I (which I was in 2008) or as a woman living with metastatic cancer presently (stage IV) without beginning with the relationships I have formed. It started in 2008 when I found a group of women through breastcancer.org and we helped each other through our treatments. We still support one other, cancer or not.

A second joy has been the ability to put more effort into my children and their activities. I am involved in my youngest daughter's dance studio and have become a mentor and teacher for musical theater. I've always had this passion but the joy of being to pass on my knowledge and watch them grow is an immeasurable pleasure.

Lastly, being able to say sometimes "I need to take to care of me first" has been an unexpected joy. This is not selfish or self-centered but rather the reality of a cancer diagnosis, and if we can really see this for what it is, our lives and the lives around us will be changed.

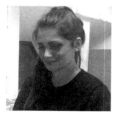

Tomorrow Will Be a New Day

BY RHONDA L SCHMIDT

"With the new day comes new strength and new thoughts."
— *Eleanor Roosevelt*

When my mother died from breast cancer, I was 12 years old and my younger brother was nine. Looking back, I can see that my father didn't know how to handle the loss of his wife and the mother of his children. None of us knew how to grieve. The days were silent, and our evenings together were beyond sad.

I remember one night when my father came into my room. I could no longer quiet my tears, the anguish was more than a pre-teen could manage. Dad held my head against his chest as I cried. I cried because I missed my mother, I cried because I was confused and scared and angry. Dad didn't say anything while I was crying, he just let me cry. After a while, I wiped my face off and at almost the same time, Dad and I said the same thing out loud.... what Mom always said to us when we were having a difficult day, "Tomorrow will be a new day." Saying it out loud with Dad brought the joy to my heart that I needed.

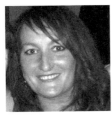

It's Independence Day

BY TONYA BOWERS

"Choose a job you love and you will never have to work a day in your life."
— Confucius

I guess I was an obnoxious child, singing at the top of my lungs to anyone within hearing distance. It didn't matter that I didn't always know the lyrics or the tune. Pull out the family albums, and there I am with my mouth wide open belting something out in almost every picture that includes me.

Twenty-two years later, I was diagnosed with breast cancer. One morning I was having trouble managing the drainage tubes and becoming angrier by the minute. The anger surprised me because I rarely get angry, but it felt as if everything in my life was getting more and more out of control. I remember looking in the mirror and wondering where me and my singing dreams had gone.

Thank goodness the house was empty because I opened my mouth and sang Martina McBride's song, *Independence Day*. It felt great! After that I started singing at churches and clubs as often as I could. My spirit soared. The joy I feel when I sing became my best healing.

Take Care of Yourself

BY PAMELA WATSON

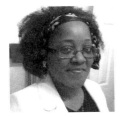

"Be gentle with yourself. You are a child of the universe, no less than the trees and the stars. In the noisy confusion of life, keep peace in your soul."
— Max Ehrmann

When I was diagnosed with breast cancer I was terrified and upset with God for interrupting my life. However, I learned to be grateful because I learned who my friends were and how important it was for me to take care of myself. I was the type who had to be at every party, somewhat a roadrunner. I am now back going to parties, but the parties that I want to attend.

I enjoy making people laugh. Laughter is what helped me get through my intense chemotherapy and radiation treatments. I'm a very joyful person and thank God daily for this second chance.

When I was told I had breast cancer, I didn't want anyone telling me anything about what God had to say until I heard my mom say "God said by His stripes we are healed... when I finally read Isaiah 53:5 and made those words personal is when I finally found comfort and believed I would be healed.

I am an advocate reminding women to take care of themselves.

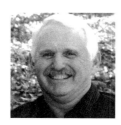

The Pain and the Gain

BY DAVID VOTE

"Gain happiness by living in the present — without regret for the past or fear of the future." — *Jonathan Lockwood Huie*

My wife and I married when we were teenagers, 42 years ago. When she was diagnosed with breast cancer in 1992, I learned to be there for her in a different way.

I learned to listen differently to her pain, her fears, and her anguish, I realized that once she was heard, really heard, she began talking more about her goals and her dreams than she did her pains and her fears. These talks were pivotal moments in our lives. Our relationship deepened, we each became stronger in this breast cancer experience. We began to trust each others' hopes and ideas for the future. Through the pain and the gain, one day turned into a week, then into months, and now we find something to celebrate every day.

We almost lost sight of the many gifts of daily life. By learning to listen more compassionately with each other, we accepted yet another unmeasurable blessing (and tool) for life.

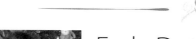

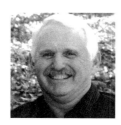

Early Detection Saves Lives

BY FRAN YOCCA

"Patience and diligence, like faith, moves mountains."
— *William Penn*

My journey began with my annual mammogram. I was called back for another "look.".. well it was cancer. During my surgeries, chemo, and reconstruction, my oncologist suggested that I talk to a geneticist, because there were no reasons for me to have breast cancer before the age of 50. They did the testing to see if I carried the BRCA gene. The test came back positive for BRCA2.

My sister went to get tested because she obviously had a 50% chance of having the same defect. My two brothers did not take the situation seriously and did not get tested. My sister did not have the gene defect thank goodness! About six months after I finished treatment, my brother called me to say that he found a lump in his breast. He went to the doctor and through testing found out that he had breast cancer as well.

My brother's doctor said that without my history, he would never have considered breast cancer in my brother's case. My brother and I both are past our five year anniversary now and doing well.

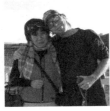

Perspective

BY AMY WU

"You must look within for value, but must look beyond for perspective."
— *Denis Waitley*

On July 23, I snapped a picture of my radiation crew alongside the radiation machine. I thanked my team with a card and a box of chocolates. It was round 15 and the end of my treatments.

The good news, life goes on, time only moves forward. I would be a case number filed away, and this chapter hopefully a memory. Soon my fellow radiation compatriots and the women who were fellow breast cancer conquerors would be in the rear view mirror. I wondered if I would forget about them. I hoped not because they have given me another perspective on life.

Not a day goes by when I don't think about cancer, either in the form of feeling grateful I am alive, contemplative of the healing process, guilty and yet elated that I am one of the survivors.

Breast cancer has changed me for the better in some ways, there is power in knowing that time is limited and not to be wasted, and in gaining perspective on people and situations.

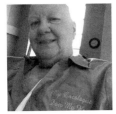

My Oncologist Does My Hair

BY CHERYL ZIBELL

"Every day is better."

I had polio when I was seven and was a diabetic my adult life. I was sure I had enough and wouldn't get cancer.

A physician's friend convinced me to get a colonoscopy and mammogram. The mammography found a lump. I chose a bilateral mastectomy without reconstruction.

I'm 68 and my husband said my boobs were not my asset. I asked him if he wanted to see them the night before surgery. He said he wasn't interested in seeing a pair of 42 longs.

My surgeon recommended a lumpectomy but I insisted on having the bilateral. With two surgeons at my side, cancer was found in my right breast and cancer in my lymph nodes in my left breast. After rechecking my tissue, the doctors concluded the bilateral mastectomy saved my life.

After the recommended medical treatments, I am doing great. Every day is better. My shirt says "My oncologist does my hair."

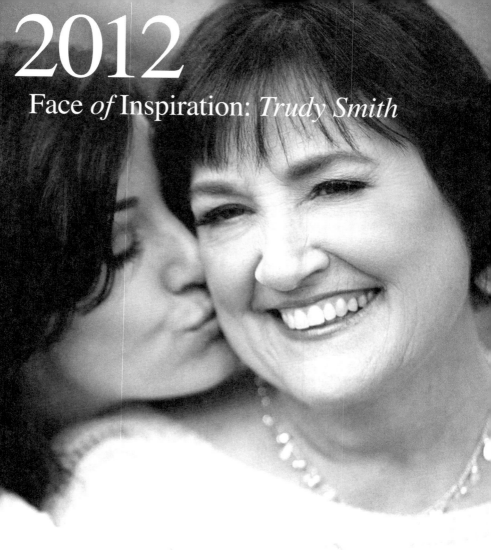

2012
Face *of* Inspiration: *Trudy Smith*

"There are miracles behind every door. Be brave enough to open one."

Be Brave

During the Face of Inspiration contest, I learned of a 70-year old breast cancer survivor who had cancer come back in her bone. Unable to save her leg, she had it amputated. I later learned that she was touched by my inspirational quote. This heart-warming experience was all the reward I needed. Participating in the Face of Inspiration contest opened a door for others to share their journey.

I chose this inspirational quote because it encapsulated my breast cancer journey. Thinking back on my breast cancer journey, I realized just how much this message of hope gave me the courage to move forward through fear, worry and anxiety. It is so hard to stay in the present. It was a challenge for everyone. I needed to repeat, one minute at a time, like a mantra. We need to show up, bravely open the door of fear, go through it and see the miracle.

I remember putting cancer behind me. It was too painful to think about those women that didn't survive. Since my journey has resurfaced through the Face of Inspiration, I find myself helping others going through the same struggle.

I've looked at fear in the eyes of many women given their diagnosis of breast cancer. Whether it is breast cancer, financial instability, divorce or grief counseling, my story has always seemed to give hope to others simply by saying that I have been a breast cancer survivor for over 25 years. Immediately they realize that anything is possible.

My motto is to trust, have courage and be brave enough to open that unknown door and go through it... the end result may be for the higher good, a miracle.

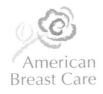

American
Breast Care

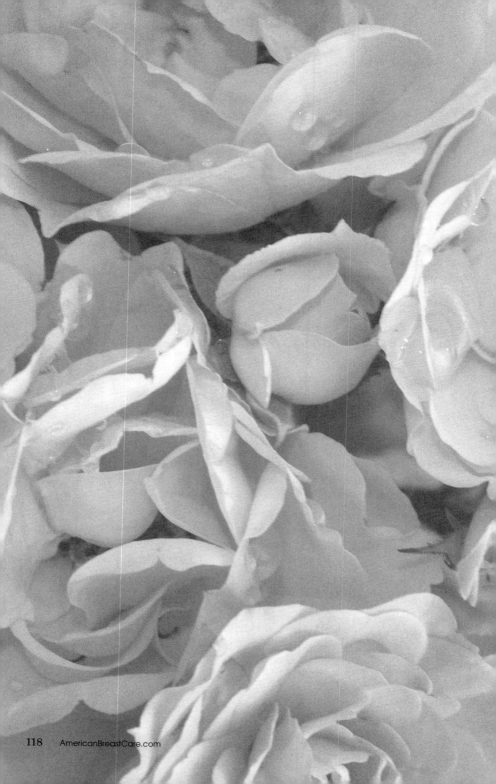

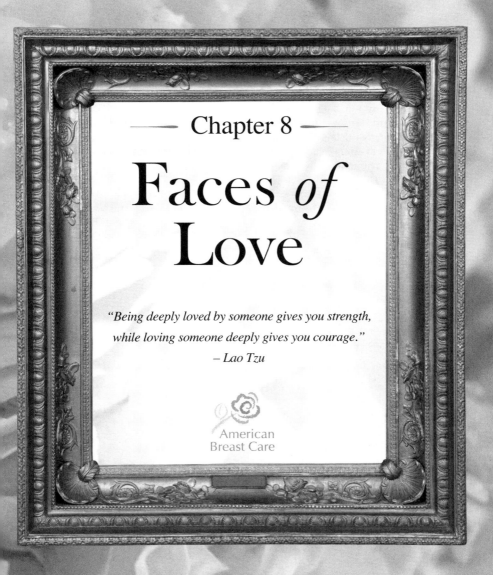

Chapter 8

Faces *of* Love

"Being deeply loved by someone gives you strength,
while loving someone deeply gives you courage."
– Lao Tzu

American
Breast Care

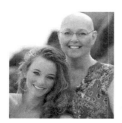

I Have Never Felt So Loved

BY KAREN ALBERT

"Love keeps us strong."

I was diagnosed with stage IIIb inflammatory breast cancer on April 23, 2013. It was so hard telling my son and daughter; I worried about how this would affect their lives. My daughter Amy was a senior in high school and we had many important events coming up! I started chemo on May 9th and my treatments affected me pretty quickly. Amy and I were used to doing everything together and I realized that our lives were going to be different for awhile. We managed to get through every event including dance recitals, prom, graduation and a graduation party with the help and love of my husband Jim and our families. It was amazing how everyone came together and made Amy's senior year a wonderful, fun experience! Amy is now at college and I have completed my bilateral mastectomy and radiation. I couldn't have made it through the past nine months without my love for my husband and children and the love from our family and friends. It has been a rough journey but I have never felt so loved. My cancer diagnosis has deepened my love for life and the people around me.

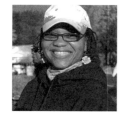

I've Gone Through the Fire

BY NADA CROWDER

"Sometimes God will deliver you from the fire, and other times will make you fireproof." — Joel Osteen

You never believe it could happen to you until it happens to you. I discovered my lump shortly after Christmas in 2006 while performing my very first shower breast exam. I was alarmed by the hardness and with further examination, the size and shape of the lump in my left breast. It immediately stirred up fear. Like many women, I put the thought of cancer far away in the back of my mind until I shared the finding with my mother and sister who convinced me to seek the opinion of a medical professional.

In early January of 2007 I was diagnosed with breast cancer. My life would and has opulently changed. I take no credit, God deserves all the glory. From the day of my diagnosis throughout living in the here and now I have witnessed the characteristics of unconditional love by my Lord, family and friends. Now I aspire to be a vessel the Lord can use to encourage and share unconditional love with women I meet who are going through their own breast cancer journey. "I've gone through the fire and come out as gold!"

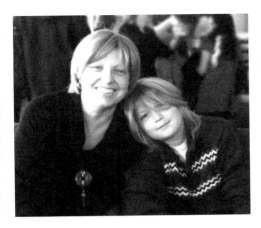

Erik's Letter

BY DONNA AND ERIK CHEFFE

"I will see you with my mom cured."

From Donna Cheffe, mother of Erik:
My son is 10 and in 5th grade. I have been stage IV for seven years and he has grown up with me fighting cancer. My son's class was given an assignment to write a persuasive letter on any topic. Most children wrote that they wanted a pet, a video game, an iPod, or longer recess. My son wrote his letter to breast cancer researchers.

Here is his letter:

October 3, 2013

Dear Cancer Researchers,
You should cure breast cancer. If you do, you will save my mom, she has stage-four breast cancer. See what benefits there are for you, and that it is a horrible sickness.

What bad things are there about having a mom with breast cancer? First of all, we spend a lot of money on chemo. I am also very worried about her. I don't know if the medicine is working. She can't do much with our family because she never feels very good.

How will you benefit from curing breast cancer? First you will make money from getting a huge bonus. You will also be famous because many people will hear about it. Most importantly you will save many lives especially my mom's.

Why is cancer a horrible sickness? First thing that makes it bad is that it ends the lives of many people every year. One of my mom's best friends died of it. She still misses her. In addition to ending the lives of many people, breast cancer also makes it hard to do things with your family and friends. Sometimes that makes friends forget about them. Another thing that makes breast cancer a horrible sickness is that it uses a lot of money to have chemo which makes it hard for some families who don't have much money.

Clearly breast cancer is a very bad sickness. My mom has stage-four breast cancer and there are many benefits for you. I will see you with my cured mom.

Sincerely,
Erik Chaffe

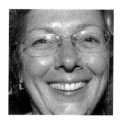

Now I See How Loved I Am

BY JEANETTE DAILEY

"The chemo made me do it."

I'm a mother of 16 year old boy/girl twins and a 12 year old daughter. In September 2010, I was diagnosed with triple negative breast cancer. It was the last thing on earth I ever thought I'd hear. After the initial shock wore off I became angry, and wanted to know why, after all my family had been thru with my mother's sudden death in 2008, why I had to get this.

You come into the world alone, but in reality you aren't alone and you touch so many peoples lives. To me this is one of the most impressive experiences I have had in my very blessed life.

I am very humbled by the love and help everyone has given to my family and me and I will always always cherish and embrace this experience. I started out angry and now I see how loved and cared for I am. Well, there is no answer as to why I got breast cancer, but there is a way to beat it, and that's what I did.

I'm a 4 year THRIVER!.

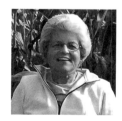

The Gift of Friendship

BY NANCY FENNO

"The greatest gift of life is friendship, and I have received it."
— Hubert H. Humphrey

My breast cancer put a temporary stop to "normal" life for my husband and me. We had been pursuing our love of wildlife photography, while traveling with our RV. We were about to head out on a trip to Vancouver Island. The trip had to be postponed so I could work on my recovery from the mastectomy and chemotherapy. I received a beautiful hand made card from my life long best friend. In the card was this poem, which Bobbie had written just for me.

The Road To Recovery
For 30 days I hope to send. A little something — to help you mend
A trinket here, a letter there. To let you know — I really care. Vancouver waits — it won't be long. Before you're singing Willie's song "ON THE ROAD AGAIN."

That was the beginning of something wonderful to look forward to every day in the mail. Each little gift came with heartfelt wishes and sometimes a good laugh that inspired me to get well. Each present was really a box filled with love from my best friend. What an inspiration!

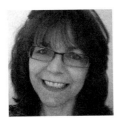

The Most Important Thing

BY COLLETTE GAUTHIER

"For me, it's all about love."

When I was diagnosed with stage IV breast cancer at the age of 46, I was told I had only 30 days to live. So, I began preparing myself for death. Not in a negative kind of way, but in a way that I found God.

I know this sounds cliché, but when you are all alone at night sweating from chemo and drugged from a fractured spine, who else is there? Or, when you are in a tube where everyone else is in a "safe" room, who is your comforter? It is easier to give up on life... to just roll over and die. So, why am I still here and what truly matters to me?

We all have to answer that question or we won't know how to truly live at all. When I am feeling weak or helpless, I pray. It is the most powerful thing I know I can do. When I am feeling blue, I do something for someone else.

For me, it's all about love. I know the day is going to pass no matter how I spend it, but some days are just meant for tea, pajamas and reruns on television.

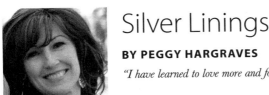

Silver Linings

BY PEGGY HARGRAVES

"I have learned to love more and forgive because I am worth it."

I have learned to love more because I am worth it.

Being in the mortgage industry for years I am pretty used to the ups and downs of it. So when I was informed that our hours were being cut at work due to decreased production I figured I would take advantage of it and get things done that I hadn't had time for. The first was to get my first mammogram. I figured at the age of 45 I was probably due, if not over due. So I set up the appointment and went and had it done.

My decision to have a mammogram was all perfect timing. I received the call at work that I had cancer. I was diagnosed with DCIS with micro invasion. After much research and discussions with the doctors I decided to go through with a bilateral mastectomy and reconstruction.

After almost 3 years and 13 surgeries later I know I am not the same person I was. I know to hate the beast but embrace the journey, for we are the leaders of our own happiness. I have learned to love more, and forgive because I am worth it. There really are silver linings in the journey if you just open your heart.

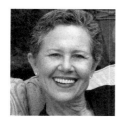

I Am Open to Receiving

BY BRENDA KAMBAKHSH

"To graciously receive is an expression of the dignity of giving."
— Deepak Chopra

I used to believe that being independent was a positive trait. I learned it is not a universal aspiration when I taught in West Africa. I asked for assistance from my African colleague in finding a seamstress, and then waited a few weeks. When she did not respond I sought a referral through other means. I did not allow her time to help me in a culture where social dependency is of primary importance. She was deeply offended and I was embarrassed.

A defining trait of Americans is independence; we are proud of it! When I was diagnosed with breast cancer, I had my attitude again, "I can do this myself." Soon after my diagnosis a survivor friend blessed me with the advice I needed, "Allow others to support you; give them that gift."

This brief statement changed my cancer journey. I opened my heart to receiving. By allowing others the joy in giving, amazing blessings appeared, often in moments of despair. Be ready to receive, always, and be nourished with love and abundance.

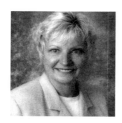

Resilience

BY LINDA KMETZ

"What lies behind us and what lies in front of us are tiny matters compared to what lies within us." — Ralph Waldo Emerson

"It's in the liver." Those words spoken by my sister Karen's oncologist sent a surge of emotion through me. Being a nurse and carrying the "burden of knowledge" I knew my sister had not only an uncertain future but a life-threatening course of chemotherapy head of her.

Before she was diagnosed with stage IV metastatic breast cancer in 2008, I would describe my baby sister as a "wimp." Being the youngest of three siblings, my parents naturally protected and indulged her (in other words, they spoiled her!). I wondered how she would be able to endure the rigors of treatment.

From her initial metastatic diagnosis to now, I see in my sister a sense of resilience, hardiness and a determination to survive that still serves as a source of inspiration to me every day. Through six rounds of chemotherapy, three recurrences, two surgeries and a hospitalization related to a serious side effect of her on-going treatment, Karen has not only worked full time but continues to design and sell her own line of jewelry.

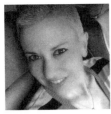

Keeping the Faith

BY CARI LANIER

"Faith is a knowledge within the heart, beyond the reach of proof."
— Khalil Gibran

One morning in February 2010 my dog jumped on my chest which caused me to feel a lump in my breast.

At the age of 33, I was told that I had breast cancer and that I needed medical treatment. I walked in a premier cancer center with my records and said "I need help!" Within an hour an oncologist saw me, ordered tests, told me I had stage IIb breast cancer and I started my first chemo treatment on March 3, 2010. I went through a left breast mastectomy in April 2010. I had the DIEP procedure and six breast reconstructive surgeries.

During chemo I stayed positive and that helped keep my spirits up along with creating a website where I shared my complete story along with photos from all of my surgeries. The website was a form of therapy for me, but it helped others by spreading inspiration and awareness.

The one thing I did was keep my faith! And that is the most valuable piece of advice I can pass forward. I am now three years cancer free!

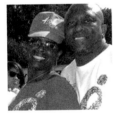

A New Reality

BY PAMELA MARTIN

"Love like never before."

I love to sing. I'm not a singer but there is always a song on my heart. The day I walked into the doctor's office and heard the words "you have cancer," my song was changed forever. I told my doctors to recheck their results — they had the wrong person. My reality was changed forever.

My new reality was having a mastectomy at the age of 34 followed by chemotherapy which introduced me to a totally new reality. I had to surrender to side effects of drugs that were meant to help me survive this disease but caused nausea, loss of hair (all of it), discomfort and night sweats.

Now, 12 years later, I am grateful for the experience. I may have lost a lot of things but what I've gained outweighs the losses. I've learned to love and love hard. I've learned to live each day as if it was my last. I've learned not to sweat the small stuff; if by God's grace I was able to defeat cancer, why should I worry about anything else?

I live by these words: LIVE like it's my last day. FIGHT like it's my last chance. LOVE like never before. By the grace of God... I AM A SURVIVOR!

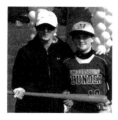

That is the Best Part

BY KELLI MERCURIO

"The giving of love is an education in itself." – Eleanor Roosevelt

I found out I had breast cancer on my son Jonathan's 10th birthday. One night after treatment Jonathan asked, "Mommy, "What is the worst part about having cancer?" I told him, "It is probably the chemotherapy. It makes me feel sick sometimes and then I can't do the things I want to do with you, like going to see your baseball games."

I wanted this to be a teachable moment, I leaned close and said, "But do you know what the best part of cancer is?" Jonathan thought for a moment and replied "Is it all the meals people are bringing us?"

I smiled and said, "Yes, look at all of the the wonderful things people are doing for us, bringing us meals, taking you to practice and to see your friends.

God never intended for us to go through anything alone. Look at how many people are surrounding us with love.

That is the best part.

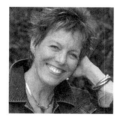

The Heart of the Matter

BY BARBARA MUSSER

"Begin doing what you want to do now. We are not living in eternity. We have only this moment sparkling like a star in our hand – and melting like a snowflake." – Marie Beynon Ray

Beyond the physical trauma of breast cancer, many women experience love trauma — self-love, romantic and sexual love and love of life. Love is the heart of the matter, and breast cancer opens the door for us to explore what love means to us.

Because our bodies change so much, it's easy to think we are no longer lovable. We can judge ourselves as less beautiful and desirable; wonder if our sexiness is gone or question if anyone will want to be intimate with us. Many women say that intimacy and sex weren't great before and now it hardly seems worth it.

Under this is the yearning to be seen, accepted and loved now. We all need to feel deeply emotionally connected and loved, and fear we may not be.

The first place to connect emotionally is with yourself — you are beautiful and lovable because you are a perfect and precious soul. When you know that you radiate beauty to the world, and that is irresistible, totally lovable.

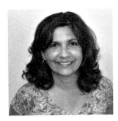

Love Heals

BY NATALIE PALMER

"We accept the love we think we deserve." — *Stephen Chbosky*

My breast cancer journey began with a lump, a prayer and a metastatic breast cancer diagnosis. At the time I had only the vaguest idea of what metastatic meant. Unfortunately, it's one of those words — once you know it, you know it for life.

Metastatic is a word I live with now. Meta, as I like to call her, and I have become old friends. We have an agreement that's been working out great for the last eight years. I agreed to love myself in every possible way by taking care of ME. She agreed to leave me alone to heal.

Now I treat myself with kindness, compassion and appreciation. I became my new best friend! I used to be critical, judgmental and a bit of a bully to myself. Nothing I did ever measured up. When I got sick I prayed for strength and guidance. Through prayer I realized I needed to stop unhealthy behaviors so that I could heal.

Today I love myself more than ever. Meta has kept her part of the agreement and I've been cancer-free for almost eight years.

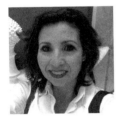

The Smallest Joys

BY DOREEN RUGGIERO

"Start doing by doing what's necessary, then do what's possible, and suddenly you are doing the impossible." — *Francis of Assisi*

My name is Doreen Ruggiero, I am 51 years old. I was diagnosed with a triple positive tumor two years ago. Like most women, I was devastated by the diagnosis. I didn't have time for breast cancer. I already had two jobs; I am a J.D. with an administrative position in the courts, and I am an adjunct professor.

I opted for a bilateral mastectomy. Because my tumor was Her2 positive, my medical team recommended chemotherapy and 52 weeks of herceptin infusions. Except for the bad taste in my mouth and nausea, I fared pretty well.

Cancer changes you, both inside and out. Suddenly you are awakened to the reality that life may be shorter than you expected. You really become grateful for the smallest joys, and you worry so much less about unimportant things.

There will be a time when the experience is just a memory. You may even come to view it as a blessing because it teaches you so much about yourself, your faith, and the support of family and friends that you may not have known otherwise.

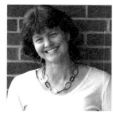

My Care Plan

BY BRITTA WILKS MCKENNA

"Do what you can, with what you have, where you are."
— *Theodore Roosevelt*

Although it took a lumpectomy, mastectomy, two reconstruction surgeries, nipple construction and areola tattoo, the long road to reconstruction was worth it for me. It was a way for me to feel whole again, to be balanced and to be able to confidently wear clothing and feel and look healthy again. I have four tips:

1. Get fit. Do what you can do at that moment. After surgery or when you are experiencing the worst of your treatments, it may be walking to the bathroom, but set a goal to make it to the end of the block. Then walk a mile and keep challenging yourself to move down the path to recovery.

2. Look your best. Don't forget to do something nice for yourself – get a massage or even just put on your lipstick to regain control and start down the road to feeling yourself again.

3. Keep your cool. Find a friend you can dump on, vent to and cry on their shoulder so you can keep your cool all the other times.

4. Ask for help. Your friends and family want to help you. Give them an opportunity to be part of your recovery plan by including them in your care circle.

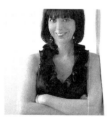

The Gifts in Cancer

BY TINA WELLS

"There are really good people out there. Let them carry you through."

My professional life was on the rise, a political career was being considered, my son was thriving and so many good friends enlivened my social life when terrible news reached me of the death of my 21 year old nephew.

On the way to his funeral, I discovered a lump on my nipple. It was cancer. The following is what I learned through my journey:

1. Our attitude is our choice.
2. Refrain from judging those who aren't there for you during cancer but rather be there for them when it's their turn.
3. There are really good people out there. Let them carry you through.
4. We are spiritual beings having a human experience. The outcomes are on Divine Time.
5. Face fear head on. Faith in God and His Word, research on what it is you fear, and baby steps toward facing that fear will make things less scary.
6. We will be challenged to do that which we think we cannot do. Count on it.
7. Cancer is actually a blessing in disguise. Stay open up to that.

A Kiss on My Bald Head

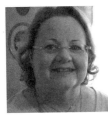

BY KIMBERLY WRIGHT

"Oh the memories... so many more good than bad."

I found my lump while in the shower on New Year's Eve 1994. So 1995 certainly started off with a bang. My daughter was two. I had just turned 36 in November.

Caitlin was my little piece of joy through it all. One of my most poignant memories of that time revolves around her bedtime. I was always careful to keep my bald head covered with at least a terry turban, pink of course.

One night as I kneeled next to her bed, I noticed her looking at it and I asked her if she might like to see what my head looked like. Caitlin nodded yes and so I slipped the turban off. She looked at my head for a moment and then reached out and placed her little hands on both sides of my head and pulled it down to her. She leaned in and placed a kiss right on my bald scalp. I heard my husband sniff behind me (bedtime was a family affair) Then she looked at me and said,"Okay, Mommy, you can put your hat back on now!" We all laughed.

Oh the memories... so many, more good than bad.

With An Open Heart

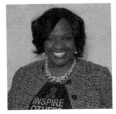

BY BETH BORDEN-GOODMAN

"Live life for purpose, on purpose and with purpose because it's THAT purpose in which you will have a life to live."

I believe I was blessed with breast cancer for others to see.

I realize daily that my diagnosis, mastectomy, reconstruction and chemo were all so not about me. It was for the purpose to bless many others — sisters, daughters, mothers and brothers.

I was selected with purpose to be a shining PINK star to brighten the paths of survivors and supporters both near and far. I 'sPrINKle' PINK on purpose and make people think not to let breast cancer make them shrink!

What a wonderful responsibility that I've been given! I've embraced it and in a wonderful shade of pink I'm living.

It came with a few bumps (new 'girls'), bruises (tram flap scar) and high-fives. It was ALL worth it — you see I'M ALIVE!

With my P.I.N.K. purpose, I have a life to live. With an open heart I freely give. I give 'sprinkles' of love, hope, courage and faith, hoping to comfort and strengthen any warrior's current state.

2011

Face *of* Inspiration: *Elizabeth Wagner*

"Each day
comes bearing
its own gifts.
Untie the
ribbons."

— Ruth Ann Schubacker

The Gifts of Life

Growing up in a small southern town, I considered myself lucky to be surrounded by my family, friends and love ones. I was the star reader of my class, a catcher for the Rivermont Elementary team and Kathy's best friend. I was blessed with loving parents; my father was strong enough to carry me on his shoulders at bed time. Truly, my childhood was a gift.

As I grew older, I learned to cope well with every day life, but breast cancer was something entirely new. When I was diagnosed with breast cancer in 1993, my immediate response to the doctor was, "You have the wrong patient's file! I'm very healthy!" How could I have stage III breast cancer at 42?

The diagnosis came swiftly, within three weeks of a 'routine' examination. However, given that the patient file was indeed mine, and I did have breast cancer at a relatively young age, I am thankful that I had my family, friends and medical community to rally around me.

As a 21-year breast cancer survivor, I am glad I get to watch my two girls grow into lovely women as well as laugh often with my husband while enjoying living life.

From my inspirational quote, I hope women gain that each day should be taken as a gift which has limitless bounds. When we receive a gift, it is often wrapped in exquisite paper, sealed with a satiny bow. It doesn't reveal its secret... it could be a cordless drill, a crayon portrait, or a lovely cashmere wrap! We gently tug the ribbons and see what is hidden within.

Sometimes we are confused, sometimes charmed and sometimes delighted by the contents! However, we have had that moment to experience the anticipation, the wonder and joy of being the recipient of a precious offering. Each day is given to us in the same manner. With a grateful heart, we receive this beautiful offering, and then we weave our hands into the ribbons of the day to see what awaits us. It could be a gorgeous sunrise, a cold medical examination, or an afternoon cup of tea with a friend. We never know what the day will hold, but we do know we are blessed to be able to slide our fingers into each of ribbons to see what the day will bring. What a gift to have the knowledge that there can be joy.

Like many in a stressful situation, it has become easy for me to slip into hopelessness and frustration. Will the treatments ever end? Will the nausea ever stop? Will I be able to work again? By focusing each day on my quote taped to the mirror, I reminded myself that I didn't know what each day held. Sometimes I knew days would hold big challenges; however, I also was reminded that there could be joy and comfort in the small pleasures. It was up to me to have faith that there could be good in each day, and to untie those ribbons to find the treasures.

It is tempting to recall a moment with my medical team and state, 'That's when I knew I would be fine!" But that was not my reality. My real pivotal moments came building on each other. First, my family was endlessly comforting, but they also reminded me that I needed to get dressed for the piano recital and share some ideas for the upcoming birthday party. Next, my moments were built by survivors who had been down this path and reached back with support and courage. They came with casseroles, took my children to the zoo and listened to my fears; they showed me the path as they had walked it and gave me real hope. Finally, my doctors reinforced these moments when they asked me to reach out to other women facing the same diagnosis. For me, the confidence of my family, friends and doctors helped me inch away from despair and gave me hope that there would be a good end to this challenge.

The Inspiration Form adds to the start of my day. My breast form now serves as a gentle reminder of all the gifts in my life like my family, friends and loved ones. Every morning, I'm greeted with an inspirational message that is carefully inscribed on the back of my breast form. Seeing this message everyday inspires me to live a fuller life. It is just that little something extra that makes me want to live, feel and inspire.

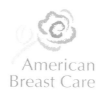

American
Breast Care

— Chapter 9 —

Faces *of* Transformation

"Nature often holds up a mirror so we can see more clearly the ongoing processes of growth, renewal, and transformation in our lives."
– *Mary Ann Brussat*

American
Breast Care

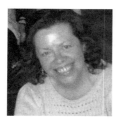

The New DonnaSue

BY DONNASUE BAKER

"We can let circumstances rule us, or we can take charge and rule our lives from within." — Earl Nightingale

If someone would have told me six years ago that life could be better after breast cancer, I know I wouldn't have believed them. When I was diagnosed with breast cancer, I was 42, going through a divorce, I had two teenage sons, and I wanted to sue my employer for "misconduct."

I probably should mention that I was bitter about my soon to be ex-husband's new girlfriend. Life was not fair at the time. My attitude, health and life changed after an elderly co-worker said to me that life isn't about fairness and to get over my woes. She said life is about learning to do something happy every day for yourself and for someone else, in spite of life's imperfections and hardships.

That was my wake-up. I stopped my complaining, got myself involved in my health needs, applied for a new job, starting hugging my boys everyday and made them hug me back. I learned to give something back everyday and told my doctors to pay better attention to my medical needs because the old DonnaSue wasn't in charge any more.

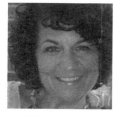

Be a Wellness Warrior

BY CONNIE CIFELLI

"Live, not just exist!"

My journey over the last five years has taken me down many roads. After my first diagnosis in 2008, I was determined to live a healthier lifestyle and transform my body. I did that by losing 70 pounds and I never felt better! This was accomplished by taking thriver programs offered by a local holistic wellness foundation. Breast cancer struck again in 2010.

This time it hit me hard on an emotional level. I could not let go of the fear that comes with a cancer diagnosis; it consumed me from head to toe. It was all I thought about every waking moment. I finally got through it with the help of amazing spiritual healer and a healing retreat offered by the holistic foundation. Through these programs I have been able to move on with life.

I believe people should "LIVE" — not just exist. My second cancer journey has brought me to a place of wellness not just for my body, but my mind and soul as well. I have refocused my life. It is not about having cancer, it is about being a WELLNESS WARRIOR!

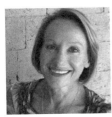

My Journey

BY GAI COMANS

"Travel is more than the seeing of sights; it is a change that goes on, deep and permanent, in the ideas of living." — Miriam Beard

The year 2000 was a magical one in Sydney, Australia, the new millennium, the Olympics in September, there were endless parties as the city was abuzz with excitement.

I was 38. My year also began as a magical one, I married my long-term love and felt like a princess. Then suddenly the magic bubble burst a few months later and after three long months of testing I was diagnosed with an aggressive form of breast cancer. My doctor gave me little chance of living through the next few years, but deep down I was determined that I would survive, and I did.

I knew to truly LIVE big, changes had to be made; I gave up my corporate executive role to work full time helping breast cancer survivors thrive post treatment and I decided to travel to the most inspiring places in the world.

My true healing after treatment came when I took action and began to experience life again, leading me to places and people that I had only ever dreamed of.

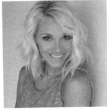

My Butterfly

BY GINA COOK

"What the caterpillar calls the end of the world, the master calls a butterfly." — Richard Bach

I was 31 years old and a mother of my two young daughters, Macayla and Dakota. Just days before my youngest daughter Dakota's first birthday, I was diagnosed with breast cancer.

Yet through it all, my heart still had a song.

I will forever remember watching my oldest daughter Macayla chasing butterflies in our front yard. Through Macayla, I was witnessing hope, joy and transformation that was calling my name.

I went into my closet, knelt down on the floor and with paper and pen birthed the song out of its' cocoon "My Butterfly."

My butterfly, you fly so high. You fly for me. Everything I am not now, you seem to be. My Butterfly take on the wind, fly so high, but come back again. Thank you for letting me see, myself through you. You're everything to me.

I began to see myself emerge from the cocoon and able to fly, not physically but spiritually. I felt real HOPE and today I have more confidence than ever before. I pray you feel the hands of God on your life.

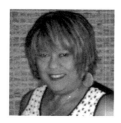

Meeting the Challenges

BY KATHIE PALADA DIXON

"My cancer scare changed my life. I'm grateful for every new, healthy day I have. It has helped me prioritize my life." — Olivia Newton-John

In March 2009, I was diagnosed with infiltrating ductal carcinoma. I was planning my 60th Birthday Celebration. This became an interruption in my life. I knew I had to be proactive with what was happening so I researched the diagnosis and my medical team.

I had a lumpectomy with 16 lymph nodes removed. I was in stage IIIa. My treatments of chemotherapy and radiation treatments took a total of nine months to complete. During this time my father died of cancer. I held tight to his example of strength to get me through.

I found a way of giving back by volunteering to help patients with their emotional support for their journeys.

On April 25th I celebrated my 65th Birthday and four years in REMISSION. I have held on to my faith in GOD and HOPE. I thank my husband for standing by me and all my family and friends. I have enjoyed retirement, writing poetry, designing jewelry, gardening and painting. I learned to clear the hurdles and meet the challenges.

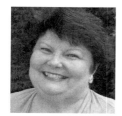

Doing What You Love

BY WENDY DOHERTY

"Life is a lot sweeter when you spend it doing what you love."

When I was first diagnosed with breast cancer, I was living a life of mediocrity. I had wanted to discover my passion and change the direction of my sails on the big ship known as Life. I had no idea how that was going to happen.

Breast cancer helped me to discover courage, strength and my voice. I summoned all three and rid my life of toxic people. Now I surround myself with nutritious people who feed my soul.

A positive outcome demands energy and positive thinking. I am one of the few who openly admit that fighting breast cancer was a rewarding experience because I learned to live my life differently.

We are not guaranteed a certain amount of time on Earth. Are we looking for quality or quantity? Breast cancer does give us a great lesson. We can take the good, bad and ugly and turn it into something powerful and purposeful.

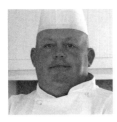

Authenticity to Life

BY CURTISS HEMM

"If you have built castles in the air, your work need not be lost; that is where they should be. Now put the foundations under them."
— *Henry David Thoreau*

I am a fan of Thoreau; his words cut to the heart of matters at hand, providing clarity of what is truly essential in my life. It turns out breast cancer does the same.

My wife's battle with breast cancer forced me to face the essence of a human life and to see the level people can, and will, rise to set a new course for living.

Breast cancer has allowed me to bear witness to the inner strength of my wife which in turn has brought an authenticity to our marriage and deepened the spiritual value and worth of our family.

Breast cancer freed me to shed the things in life that offer no return, that weigh down my emotional and physical progress and that disrupt the essence of living. I live my life with an honest, authentic and real concentration. I build relationships and not work off of transactions. In everything I seek long term success, not short term gains.

Breast cancer has given me this. For that I am thankful and blessed.

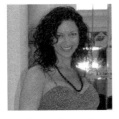

A Second Chance, Enjoy It!

BY BRIONY JENKINS

"Life is not measured by the number of breaths we take, but by the moments that take our breath away." — *Maya Angelou*

For so long, I was afraid to hope that life would feel normal again and where breast cancer wouldn't invade every waking moment of my life. I couldn't imagine a time where I would feel safe, where fear of a recurrence didn't shake my thoughts and emotions.

But that day did come, though it took a while. It crept up on me until one day I realized that my breast cancer journey had become an integral part in making me who I am today. Breast cancer took so much but in its way, it gave so much too.

To survive is a second chance at life, an opportunity to embrace every day and to value the possibility of growing old from a whole new perspective. It is feeling blessed to be alive; humbled by acts of love and kindness from friends, family and even total strangers. Yes, we have scars, but they are symbols of our courage and triumph over cancer.

To be able to say "I am a Survivor" is truly a gift, enjoy it!

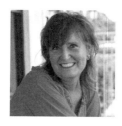

It Was Time

BY HEATHER JOIE

"Laugh often."

Ten years after I was diagnosed with breast cancer I started my own business designing and making lingerie for breast cancer survivors. I struggled with the disfigurement and scars. I met so many other women who had these same issues. It was tough to feel sexy, and even tougher to find fun, sexy, and flattering nightgowns.

After three lumpectomies and finally a mastectomy, loss of hair from chemo, and all the other stuff that comes with cancer, I decided that to help me through it all I would be happy, laugh often, and take more risks.

I had just moved to a new city with no family and no friends, and three months later I was told that I had breast cancer. I got comfortable in the job, worked there for eight years, and forgot about the take more risk promise that I made myself. Then I was visiting a friend on her death bed. It was time. The next day I started my business, took all my savings and investments, and proudly make the garments in USA. I am very happy and laugh often!

Live with Expansive Joy

BY LONI KAPLAN

"Life is not about waiting for the storm to pass. It's about learning to dance in the rain." — Vivian Greene

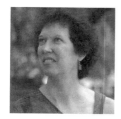

A year after I was diagnosed with lung cancer, and a year before I was diagnosed with breast cancer, I began to dance. Following the YMCA Livestrong program, I was strong enough. One year after I had been in the hospital getting a biopsy, I was in North Carolina doing contra dancing for a week, seven hours each day. I had never danced before, and was amazed that my body not only had the strength and energy to dance that long, but that I was good at it, and enjoyed it.

I live my life joyfully, and have encouraged others to live with expansive joy. I continue to travel, including a memorable trip last summer with my children to Newfoundland.

Just like my blue eyes, cancer is a part of who I am, but it does not define me. Friends have told me how my positive attitude has influenced them to more fully enjoy life, by driving with the windows down, savoring a meal with family or reading on a hammock at sunset.

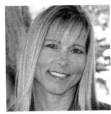

Taking Care of Me

BY ANGELA LONG

"I have come to believe that caring for myself is not self indulgent. Caring for myself is an act of survival." — Audre Lorde

I was only 35 and a mother to my two year old daughter and my five year old son when diagnosed with breast cancer in 2004. Desperate to survive to see them grow up, I closely followed doctors' orders. I was more of a spectator than an actor in my own care.

After treatment ended and the doctors' work was done, I felt like a ticking time bomb waiting for my cancer to return. Rather than explode emotionally, I used that anxiety as the fuel I needed to take an active role in my survivorship and my journey toward thrivership.

I learned how to take better care of my body through nutrition and exercise, how to choose my thoughts carefully, to listen to my spirit, and reach for my dreams and goals. I became my own advocate and in the process my journey has led me to empower others to advocate for themselves.

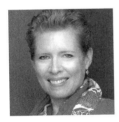

Think Differently

BY MOLLY MACDONALD

"Don't run from tests and hardships. As difficult as they are, you will ultimately find joy in them; if you embrace them, your faith will blossom under pressure and teach you true patience as you endure. And true patience brought on by endurance will equip you to complete the long journey and cross the finish line—mature, complete, and wanting nothing." — James 1:2-4, The Voice (VOICE) version

In April 2005, I received a call from my OB/GYN who had delivered all five of my children, delivering what for 40,000 women a year in this country, is a death sentence!

While my early stage disease was not about to take my life, it did take my livelihood.

Within weeks, without any income, our family faced real financial hardship. My attempts to get help were met with blank stares. It was then, under great pressure, claiming my faith, I began to think differently. *What if I could give help?*

That single change from *getting* to *giving* gave me the endurance, patience and joy I needed to not only finish treatment, but to embrace another journey altogether. One that has matured me, completed me, and left me wanting one thing, to make a REAL difference in the lives of breast cancer survivors.

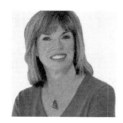

I Became What I Wanted

BY ALICE MCCALL

"There is always a gift inside."

In 2007 lightening struck and rocked my life. I was diagnosed with breast cancer — ductile carcinoma. I was fearful despite being a healing facilitator.

I worked on releasing my fears and then something wonderful happened. I felt divinely guided on how to proceed. Support resources and information which were paramount to my healing, came to me as I needed them. My connection to God was closer and more intimate than ever before.

My journey changed from focusing on healing a health issue to learning how to really live in trust — knowing that all is in divine, perfect order.

I was guided to release old buried wounds from deep in the cells of my body. I became so light and bright that people could not believe that I was in the middle of a healing process for breast cancer.

I became what I wanted — a whole, healthy, and spiritually aligned person.

Now seven years later, I continue to master my fears, live in trust, and follow the wisdom and guidance of my heart. This was my gift — a new way to live in spiritual alignment.

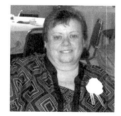

Two Choices That Day

BY RITA MIRACLE

"When we do the best that we can, we never know what miracle is wrought in our life, or in the life of another." — Helen Keller

I had worked for 15 years with breast cancer survivors as a prosthetic fitter. You would think that I would have been better prepared when I was diagnosed with breast cancer. I decided I had two choices that day: I could wallow in self-pity and become a victim of this cancer or I could become a fighter and push through what had to be done to try and save my life. With the help of God and my family, I chose the latter.

I tried to look for the positives as I went through treatment. I had the oddest sense of humor about my experience. Oh, the stories I could tell that made me laugh out loud; from my two-year old grandson pulling my turban off my head to proudly showing everyone his bald grandma, to going to work without my boobs because my husband misplaced them the night before.

I learned many lessons through my experience with cancer. I gained humility, patience, strength, and so much more appreciation for life. I now volunteer to be an encourager for breast cancer survivors. I listen and I share information. I am a prayer warrior and a grateful survivor.

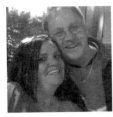

Every Step of the Way

BY LISA MIZER

"If you have only one smile in you, give it to the people you love."
— Maya Angelou

Breast cancer, the most dreaded words for women.

It was just before Valentine's Day when I was diagnosed and what a Valentine I received... February 14th was the day of my first biopsy!

Luckily, I was probably the strongest one in the family, except for my father, who promptly said, "You will get through this and we will be with you every step of the way!" He then did as he always did, he stayed strong for me.

I am thankful for my family who drove me to my various appointments and who encouraged me every step of the way. April Fool's Day was my lumpectomy, Halloween I finished my chemotherapy and on New Year's Eve my port was removed. I thank God every day that it was me and not one of my girls or my mother. It is now Valentine's Day again and I thank God every morning my feet hit the floor because I am still going strong and still cancer-free and that is the best Valentine I could ever receive. Godspeed.

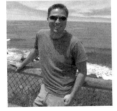

We Met in the Hallway

BY THOMAS MONDAY

"I know what love is." — *Forrest Gump*

One morning I was late to work and rushed back to the bedroom to see if I had left my keys on my nightstand. My wife Terri was carrying a load of laundry. We ran into each other in the hallway. I spilled my coffee and she dropped her basket. I helped her pick the basket back up while apologizing for being so clumsy. I saw she was crying but I also saw the scared look in her eyes.

At that precise moment in time, I felt how alone she was. Since being diagnosed with breast cancer, Terri had kept to herself, even during the effects of chemotherapy and surgery. I thought it was her way of dealing with the medical treatments. What did I really know what she was feeling; I had never asked her. Life changed that day in the hallway.

For the next two hours Terri talked, I listened. You can learn a lot by giving the floor to someone to share their vulnerabilities, their fears, their unspoken hopes. You can also re-learn what love is.

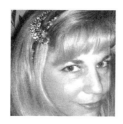

A Journey of Self Discovery

BY LINDA HILZEN MORSE

"We teach what we need most."

Breast cancer took me by surprise, 16 years ago, one month before my 41st birthday. My cancer journey did not strengthen my 19 year marriage, which was failing due to my husband's progressive mental illness that he refused to seek help for. Subsequently I was left to battle this on my own while assuming responsibility for my 14 year old daughter and nine year old son.

However, I was not alone. God's presence was with me and He put people in my life to assist me. Breast cancer took me on a healing journey of self-discovery and enabled me to nurture and care for myself. It led me to my life's work and fulfilling purpose. I have pursued a doctoral education in occupational therapy, specialized certifications in lymphedema treatment, oncology rehabilitation, and the Healthy Steps therapeutic dance program. In addition, I have become proficient as a belly dance performer and instructor. Belly dancing is empowering and embodies the feminine spirit, promoting healing, self-acceptance, and serves as a creative expression of emotions that may be difficult to verbalize. Through therapy and dancing, I teach what I most needed to learn while assisting other survivors in their own healing journey.

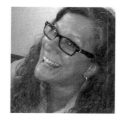

Onward and Upward

BY BONNIE PARIDAEN, MPS, RSW

"Trust your instincts."

Unbeknownst to me, breast cancer's tentacles established a secure hold into my athletic body. Fortunately, my psyche exposed the threat in a dream. It revealed a black ball in the upper left quadrant of my right breast. Somehow, I harnessed the ability to travel toward it, as though through an atomic force microscope. As the ball came into focus, it transformed from a tight round sphere into a mass of entangled, writhing snakes. They were alive and clearly on the move. The dream's message was "the snakes must be cut out."

The next year consisted of several surgeries and treatments and a load of chemo brain. As a result, I felt compelled to return to the university to exercise my foggy brain into shape. The self-reflective assignments developed into a passion toward writing a thesis on my encounter with breast cancer about illness and the shadow side of positive thinking. I graduated with a Masters in psychotherapy and spirituality and currently work as a mental health therapist.

Trust your instincts. They're here to walk alongside and guide us.

Good Things to Come

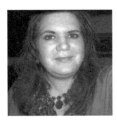

BY KATIE PARKER

"For I know the plans I have for you," says the LORD. "They are plans for good and not for disaster, to give you a future and a hope.
– Jeremiah 29:11

My very first mammogram determined that I had breast cancer. At age 36, this was the shock of my life. I had a mammogram because it was free and I like free things, even though it was against my primary care doctor's advice. Cancer wasn't what I expected or wanted, as I had no family history or palpable lump, but gave me a purpose I never had before. I felt empowered to educate others on the importance of early detection and risk factors. My cancer was caught very early.

For treatment, I had a partial mastectomy followed by six weeks of radiation. I did not meet the criteria for chemotherapy. Now at age 40, I'm not only surviving, but thriving. No matter your age, you can thrive too by becoming an active part of your treatment, finding a support group, journaling and putting your faith in a higher power. Before my diagnosis, I thought cancer would be the end. I now know that it's just the beginning of good things to come.

Thriving is Elegant

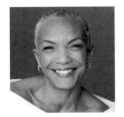

BY RHONDA SMITH

"Surviving is important. Thriving is elegant." – Maya Angelou

In May of 2008 I was diagnosed with breast cancer. There was no manual, prescription, or remedy to help me recover from the physical, emotional, and mental impacts of the experience, nor help me restore myself back to normal, whatever that may be.

Overcoming the after effects of treatment was more difficult for me than what I endured going through it. Getting my life back to what I knew as "normal" was a challenge but I soon discovered that my previous life did not promote a very healthy lifestyle.

So, I reinvented my life and priorities and now my "new normal" is about living my life with greater intention and focusing on optimizing my health and wellness. I now feel empowered to take control of my life instead of it controlling me, and I feel physically, mentally, emotionally and spiritually stronger than ever.

In my battle with breast cancer, I chose to be victorious rather than be a victim. I strive to live my life in a way that is full of vitality and without fear, so that overcoming breast cancer continues to be a life-enhancing, rather than a life-limiting, event.

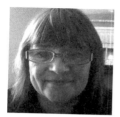

Radical Transformation

BY CINDY L YOUNG

"What doesn't kill you makes you stronger." — *Friedrich Nietzsche*

My favorite inspirational quote is "What doesn't kill you makes you stronger." Since my walk with breast cancer beginning in 2008 I have overcome many challenges. I have survived multiple surgeries, a divorce and am working to reassemble my new life as a "survivor."

I have been transformed in many ways and on many levels including spiritually, mentally, and physically.

I know that I can no longer put everyone and everything in front of my own needs for that will bring me to the depths of illness once again. I am excited to rock my new life having survived the terrible storm that breast cancer brought to my door.

Blessings to all who fight this battle for it is the fight of a lifetime!

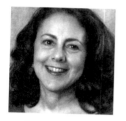

Who Would Have Thought?

BY HARALEE WEINTRAUB

"Hard times always lead to something great." — *Betsey Johnson*

I never thought my experiences with cancer would help me so much in my future life, but they did. The resolve I used to get through my cancer treatments I funneled into my post cancer personal and professional life.

The resolve I set in my mind to see my treatments through to the end, I use in meeting deadlines. The resolve I committed to make changes in exercise and diet recommended by my oncologist has made me stronger. The resolve I used to keep my sense of humor gets me through hectic days. The resolve I used to keep the big picture in mind keeps me focused on my future. These resolves helped me become fearless of new experiences, so fearless that I became an entrepreneur. Cancer gave me the strength to pursue a professional legacy and a new career. Who would have thought?

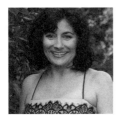

He Will Direct Your Path

BY MISSY HENSLEY

Trust in The Lord with all your heart and lean not on your own understanding. In all thy ways acknowledge Him and He will direct your paths.
— Proverbs 3:5-6

Prior to my diagnosis of breast cancer at 38 if someone had suggested playing a word association game using the letter "c", words like chocolate, crayons, cars chocolate, clouds, carnivals, and chocolate would have easily come to mind. However, when one hears the word cancer spoken in reference to their well being, the word association takes on a whole new perspective.

Proverbs 3:5-6 has always been a cornerstone in my life. At the time of my diagnosis my husband and I had a six year old daughter and a four year old son. I chose a radical approach which included a mastectomy and modified chemotherapy. Although there have been a couple of scares over the years I can say taking that course of action was the best choice. I have been cancer free for 17 years. I'm not saying that I always understand the steps my life has taken but I can say that I trust The One who I believe guides my path.

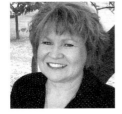

If Not Now, When?

BY BEVERLY VOTE

"Do what makes you happy." — Bernie Siegel, M.D.

Do what makes you happy isn't the usual type of prescription that a medical doctor hands out but it gave me cause to pause and rethink how I was living whatever time I have.

It would take a decade for me to learn the healing value of being happy, which is a long and unnecessary time to give that type of power over to a disease. I thought I was happy chasing the American dream and living my life by the social and marketing agendas of others. It turns out I was just busy living up to others' expectations for my life and aptly justifying my choices of unhappiness.

When I learned being happy raises endorphins and the body's immune system and states of overwhelm, despair and fear drain the body's natural energies and defenses, I made it a ritual to do something every day that makes me happy. Choosing to be happier immediately revitalized me and gave me a sense of control again.

When I ignore my options to be happier in any given moment, I ask myself if not now, when?

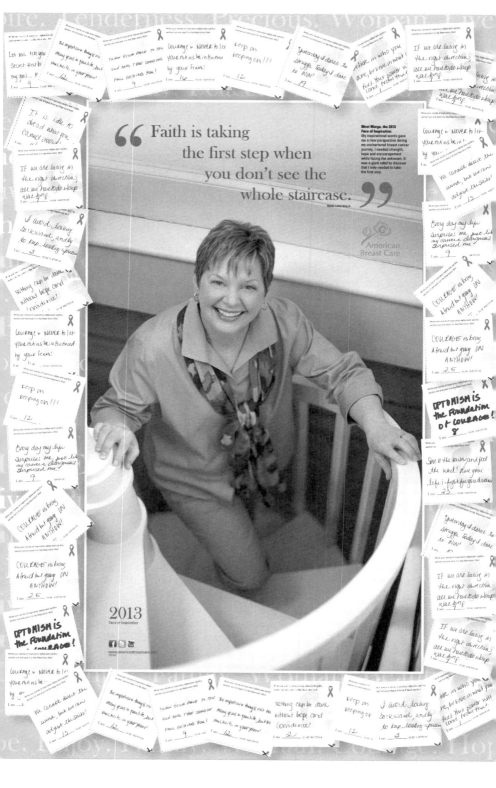

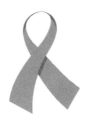

Who knows, *you* could be the next
Face of Inspiration

In honor of Breast Cancer Awareness month, American Breast Care partners with retailers across the U.S. giving breast cancer survivors the chance to participate in our annual *Face of Inspiration Contest*. This contest allows a breast cancer survivor to have a once in a lifetime experience.

It's simple to enter.

Here's how. Each fall, participating retailers display the *Inspiration Wall Poster* in a prominent area of their store for survivors to see. Survivors are asked to share and post their favorite inspirational quote on the *Inspiration Wall Poster* for a chance to win the *Face of Inspiration Contest*.

At the end of the year, participating retailers nominate a survivor to be the next *Face of Inspiration*. After reviewing all of the nominations, American Breast Care selects three finalists. Once the finalists are notified, the public is invited to vote via www.americanbreastcare.com for the woman most deserving of the *Face of Inspiration* title. This experience includes an all-expenses paid trip for her and a guest to American Breast Care's headquarters in Atlanta, GA. In addition, she will receive a special spa session, photoshoot complete with hair, makeup and wardrobe stylists, and so much more!

If you want to participate in this year's *Face of Inspiration Contest*, visit www.americanbreastcare.com/retailer.html to locate a retailer near you.

---

*The **Inspiration Wall Poster** serves as a gathering place where survivors can share and post inspirational words of hope, joy and encouragement. By creating a place where survivors can gather, we hope that many will embrace the journey of others and the power of inspiration.*

Stay Connected with ABC!

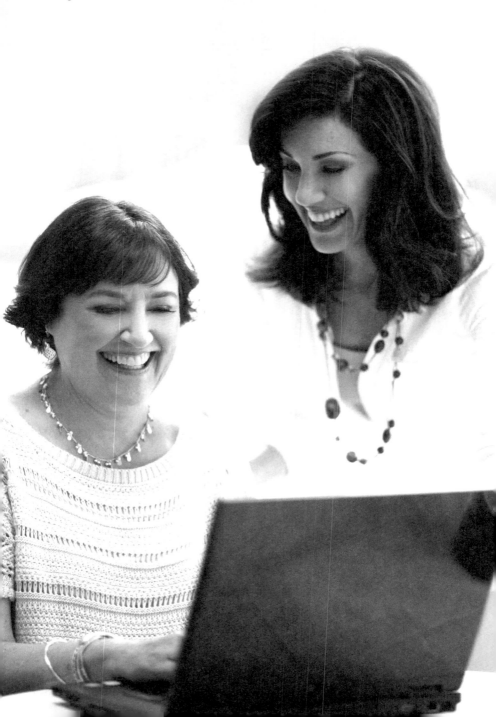

ABC wants to keep you current on the latest ABC bras and breast forms. It's important to us that you know what's available to you. Colors and styles change every season and you never know what your next favorite bra or breast form will be. We will only email you when there are new product arrivals available to you.

Ready to become an ABC Facebook fan? It's easy, visit www.facebook.com/AmericanBreastCare to "LIKE" our page.

Are you an avid "pinner"? Great! We are too! Check our boards on Pinterest. Visit American Breast Care on Pinterest at www.pinterest.com/ambreastcare.

American Breast Care has insightful and inspirational videos for you to watch via Youtube. Subscribe to the American Breast Care's Youtube channel for the latest videos. Visit www.youtube.com/user/americanbreastcare/videos.

Want to get tweets from ABC? Follow us on Twitter. Visit www.twitter.com/AmBreastCare.

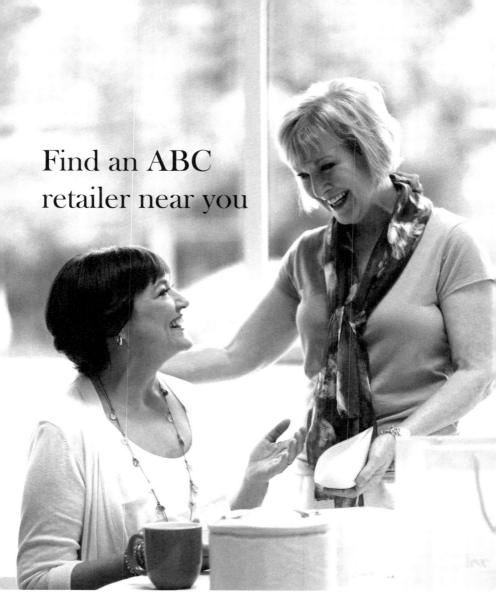

Find an ABC retailer near you

To find a retailer near you visit, www.americanbreastcare.com/retailers.html or scan QR code with your mobile device to find a retailer in your area.

After Your Breast Surgery
Know what products are available to you

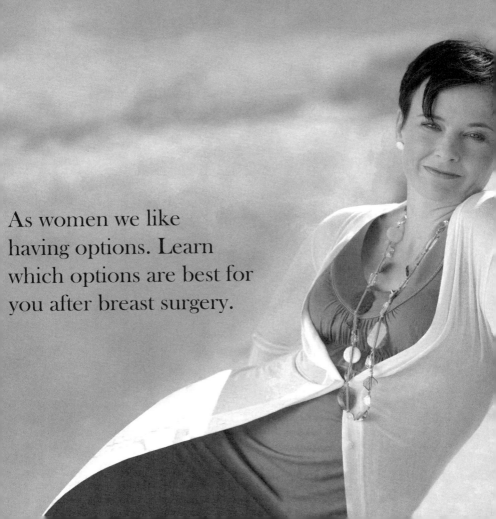

As women we like having options. Learn which options are best for you after breast surgery.

Immediately following breast surgery

Be Prepared.

Make your recovery comfortable and simple. Prior to breast surgery, ask your certified fitter about which post-surgical solutions may be the best fit for you.

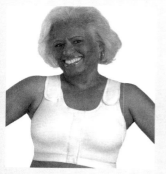

119 | Velcro Front Compression Bra

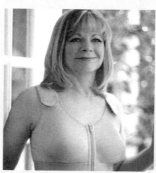

519 | Compression Bra

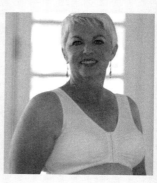

940 | Soft Bra and Form

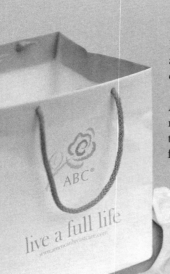

Post-Surgical Kit

Before your breast surgery, make or schedule an appointment with your certified mastectomy fitter to explore all of your post-surgical needs.

ABC's Post-Surgical Kit helps simplify your post-surgical recovery. It includes a comfortable cotton Leisure Bra, two Velcro attachable pouches for drain bulbs and a featherweight, non-silicone puff form.

6 weeks to 6 months

Be Beautiful.

Try these easy on, easy off bras for ultimate comfort and support. Consider wearing a bra with a front close adjustment or one with seamless molded cups.

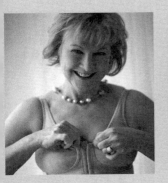

123 | Front Close Rose Contour Bra

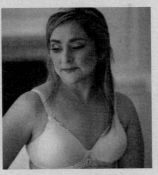

105 | Petite T-Shirt Bra

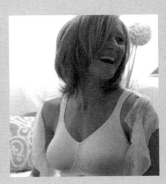

505 | Soft Shape Bra

Silicone Breast Forms

Wearing a silicone breast form offers women a non-surgical solution for restoring balance to your chest wall after a mastectomy.

A silicone breast form is usually recommended after a doctor's release. It can often be replaced every two years. Check with your insurance provider for details.

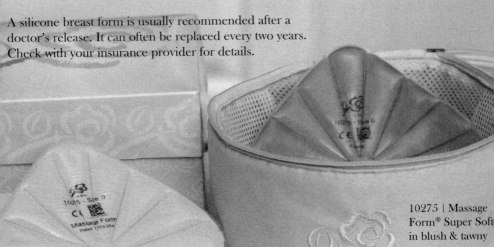

10275 | Massage Form® Super Soft in blush & tawny

All of our breast forms are made in the USA.

6 months and beyond

Be You.

Don't wait another day. Start living a fuller life today. Find a bra style and fit that suits you best!

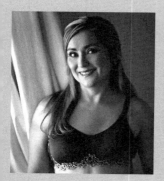

502 | Adore Bra

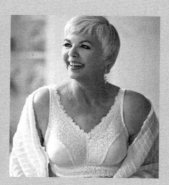

503 | Embrace Bra

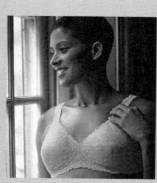

504 | Dream Lace Bra

Shapers, Partials & Enhancers

After a breast conserving surgery such as a lumpectomy, you may find that you need a shaper, partial or enhancer to restore balance and symmetry to your chest wall.

A shaper may be the right solution for you. Shapers can be worn with a pocketed or non-pocketed bra and are designed in different shapes, thicknesses and sizes to accommodate a variety of fitting needs.

Shapers, partials and enhancers are usually covered after a breast conserving surgery. Check with your insurance provider for details.

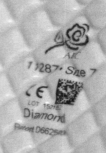

11287 | ABC Diamond Shaper Lightweight

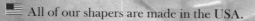 All of our shapers are made in the USA.

Gift a book to a friend!

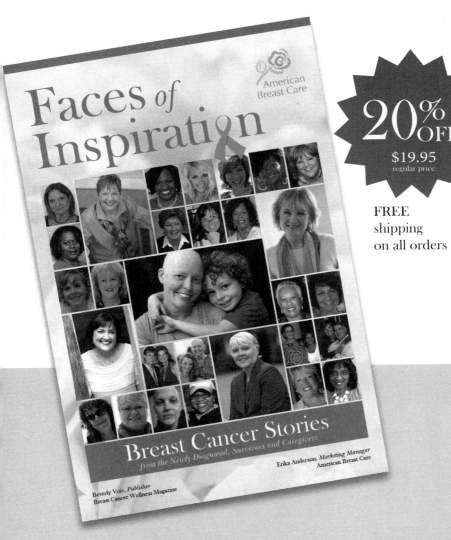

Get <u>20%</u> off regular price until Oct. 31, 2014.
Visit www.americanbreastcare.com
to purchase your copy today.

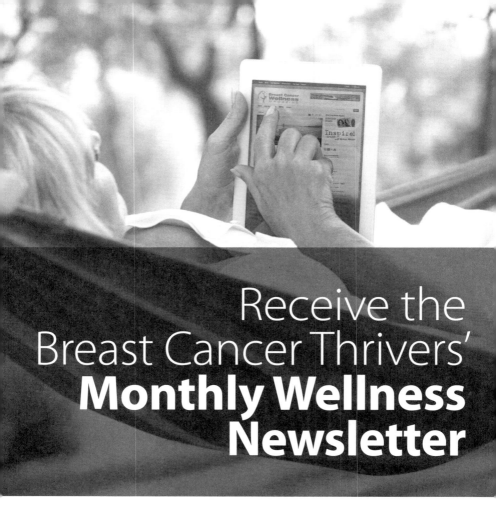

Receive the
Breast Cancer Thrivers'
Monthly Wellness Newsletter

It's free and easy to sign up!

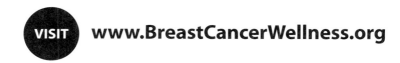

VISIT **www.BreastCancerWellness.org**

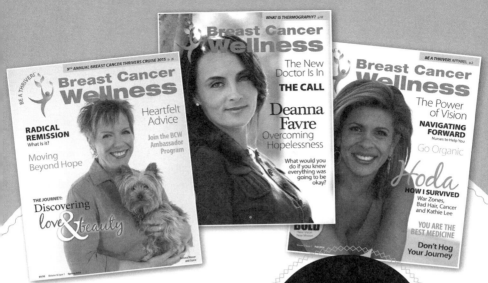

Subscribe to BCW today!

Only $15 for 1 full year

"To survive is our starting point. To thrive is our original design."

— *Beverly Vote*

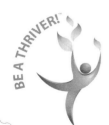

Breast Cancer Wellness

BE A THRIVER!

www.BreastCancerWellness.org

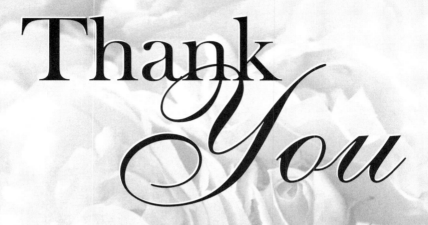

Thank You

American Breast Care
and
Breast Cancer Wellness Magazine
send a huge thank you to
all of those who opened their
hearts to share their journey
with the world.

Index